It's All in the Delivery

Improving Healthcare Starting with a Single Conversation

A Guide to Enhancing the Patient Experience Through Better Communication

---

Anthony J. Orsini, D.O.

West Essex Press
Orlando, Florida
www.westessexpress.com

© 2020 Anthony Orsini, D.O.
All Rights Reserved
Printed in the United States of America

To protect privacy, all patients' and some doctors' names have been changed. The names of Dr. Cunningham, Dr. Banks, Dr. Hernandez, Dr. Winthrop, Dr. Jones, and Dr. Patel are fictitious. All other physician names are real and have been used with their permission. For those who preferred anonymity, only first or last names were used. The name of Andia and Keith Kolakowski are real and their names and story are used with their written consent to help with their fundraising efforts.

Library of Congress Cataloging-in-Publication Data
Orsini, Anthony
It's All in the Delivery / Anthony Orsini

ISBN 978-1-09830-447-8 (paperback)

Table of Contents

A quick note:

The term "healthcare professional" is used frequently throughout this book. The comfort and healing of patients and families requires a team approach, and each medical provider is an essential component of the overall patient experience and outcome. The term healthcare professional includes anyone who directly cares for patients and families, such as, but not limited to, physicians, nurses, practitioners, physician assistants, and therapists. Regardless of the label, each is vital to the physical and mental well-being of patients and their families, and each must be skilled at communicating with compassion and forming relationships.

It's All in the Delivery, BBN P.R.O.G.R.A.M, BBN and The Orsini Way are registered trademarks of Anthony Orsini, LLC*

Dedication

This book is dedicated first and foremost to my wife Lauren, who has believed in me from the very start. Without her guidance and support, I would not have been able to continue pursuing my passion for medicine and communication training. I am eternally grateful to her for tolerating the many hours she spent alone while I worked in the NICU or traveled out of town to teach. If it were not for her words of encouragement when I was tempted to give up, this book would have never been completed.

This book is also dedicated to my children, Joseph, Summer, and TJ, for understanding that the days I spent away from home while teaching was for a greater good. In the process, I hope to have taught them the value of hard work and perseverance.

Finally, I dedicate this book to my parents who, without much means, made sure that I received the best education and medical care possible. Without their support, I have no idea where I would be today.

Special Thanks

There are so many people who are responsible for making this book a reality. In no particular order:

To the doctors of Thomas Jefferson University Hospital and

Christiana Medical Center, who took the time to mentor me and, in the process, shaped who I am as a physician. I am extremely fortunate to have had such positive role models.

To Dr. Anthony Merk, who taught me how to be a genuine person and a friend to my patients and families.

To Dr. Karen Hendricks-Muñoz, who taught me that effective leaders bring out the best in those around us.

To the real Dr. Cunningham whose tears of compassion profoundly affected me in a positive manner.

To Dr. Mary Ann LoFrumento, who gave me the chance to do my very first "Breaking Bad News" program after so many people said no. If not for Dr. LoFrumento's words, "Let's just do it and ask permission later," my dream would have never started.

To Cheryl Galante and Bob Lukasik of Bleu Moon Production and Lloyd Productions. To all the actors who dedicated so many hours crying on video to make the scenes realistic. To Chip Prestera, Joy Kigin, Sallie Glaner, Jim Serrano, Winston Haynes, Sheryl Carbonell, and all of the other actors, I am deeply grateful.

And to Maybelle Cowan-Lincoln, who not only cried on camera with the rest of the actors but also helped me get this book started. Without Maybelle's encouragement and initial edits, this book would have stopped after just a few paragraphs.

To the many volunteers who helped me teach communication skills to thousands of healthcare professionals over the past 10 years, your dedication to improving the way healthcare is delivered is greatly appreciated.

To Fred Garth and Kerrie Allen, who used their exceptional editing skills to make this book read well.

And finally, to Elizabeth Poret-Christ, who believed in what I set out to do so much that she quit her job to help me train healthcare professionals to effectively communicate and build positive relationships with patients and families. Liz's unyielding dedication and loyalty to the cause has kept this dream going. Any positive impact from this book or the teaching programs we provide is largely due to her expertise and hard work.

Prologue

Healthcare is a multi-trillion dollar industry, and the costs are steadily increasing. Advances in medicine have led to state-of-the-art diagnostic tools and new procedures that were unimaginable just a few decades ago. Cure rates for diseases such as cancer continue to rise, and new medications are being developed and introduced at a rapid pace. As the cost of more sophisticated treatments increases, medical providers are forced to compete for the limited amount of healthcare dollars that exist. The response has been an increased emphasis on efficiency and volume—often at the expense of the human interaction that is so vital to healing.

But with competition comes choice, and today's patient has more control of their healthcare than ever before. The availability of patient satisfaction surveys and internet rating/review systems provides patients with the information necessary to make a more informed decision regarding which medical provider to choose. The patient-provider paradigm is shifting from the authoritarian physician dictating treatment to a patient, to one based on a trusting relationship between two people centered around mutual respect. Therefore, a provider's ability to communicate well is more important than ever. Clinical expertise is assumed, and today's patient places a higher emphasis on a doctor's or nurse's interpersonal skills than ever before.

This evolution has compelled doctors, who otherwise might

not have placed a high priority on bedside manner, to be more personable or suffer bad reviews and a failing practice. Yet, traditionally, physicians and nurses have not been trained to be good communicators. Communication skills are not emphasized during medical training, and while some seem to be naturally adept at connecting with their patients, others find themselves struggling.

I wrote this book for healthcare professionals who want to learn communication techniques that will help them better connect with their patients, build loyalty, and express their natural compassion that attracted them to medicine in the first place. For the non-medical person—the patient who is unhappy with the impersonal, fragmented healthcare they are receiving—this book will hopefully empower you to seek out medical providers and facilities that understand medicine is about human interactions and not just about the latest, most sophisticated procedures.

For me, working to improve my communication skills did not happen because of the rise of internet reviews. It's been a career-long pursuit. In fact, this book is a compilation of 30 years of experience with thousands of doctors, nurses, and hospital staff. It represents something that I've wanted to do for a long time and, as I imagine most writers do, I would intermittently pick it up, write a few pages, and then put it down when other projects became more urgent. For that reason, it has taken longer to complete than I had hoped. However, the time and energy have finally paid off and I'm pleased with the results. I'll be even happier if this helps healthcare professionals to be better communicators and patients to better navigate an often complex healthcare system.

This book is mostly about my core passion for almost three decades: effective and compassionate communication in medicine. The art of human communication has fascinated me since I was a child. Why is one person immediately liked by people and others fail to form relationships? Why does one doctor have a thriving practice with loyal patients while others with equal clinical skills get bad reviews and struggle to build a practice? I guess it was natural that, as a physician, I was immediately drawn to studying how healthcare providers communicate, or fail to communicate with patients and with each other.

The first hurdle in writing this book was to think of a name. It had to be pertinent but also clever— a name that people would remember. There were so many suggestions and I had many great ideas that flew through my mind while driving on the interstate (driving is when I do my best thinking). One day, while coming home from a long shift, the choice became obvious, "It's all in the delivery."

Of course, I thought. Rarely does a week go by that I don't use this phrase. It applies to so many situations. I use this concept when discussing a baby's condition with a parent, convincing one of my teenagers to spend time with the family or go to church, and yes, even when persuading my wife that the shiny, new sports car I want is worth the extra money. It is the essence of communication. How we deliver the message means everything and it is the key to forming relationships, getting our point across, or showing compassion.

I first heard the phrase many years ago when I read about a famous comedian. He was asked why his jokes were always so funny. He answered, "It's all in the delivery." No matter what the situation, it is the most important rule of communicating. How we say things is just as important as what we say, if not more important. Good comedians and sales people know that how they deliver a line can be the difference between success and failure. In medicine, the stakes are even higher. There are right and wrong ways to communicate with patients and families. Whether a physician is delivering a life-changing diagnosis to a patient or family or simply meeting them for a routine visit, the method of communication is the foundation for building a relationship. Doctors and other healthcare professionals, unfortunately, are often clueless about communication techniques. We are taught that substance is more important than style. At some point, I'm sure we've all heard, "I'd rather have a good doctor with a bad bedside manner than a bad doctor with a good bedside manner." While that may be true, somewhere down the line we need to ask why we can't have both.

I am not crazy enough to compare a doctor giving tragic news to a comedian's joke or a salesman trying to sell a new car. But in medicine, more than any other profession, words matter. In fact, the ability of a healthcare professional to form relationships with patients is the number one predictor of patient loyalty. And forming relationships, as we all know, is all about communication. It is so important in medicine that studies have shown that the manner in which a physician interacts with a patient or family during a difficult conversation can affect them for decades. That's an incredible responsibility, yet medical education fails to train us in this critical skill.

The good news is that effective and compassionate communication is not hard to learn. And so, I have dedicated this book to examining, developing, and discussing these topics. If you are in the medical field, the topics that are addressed will help make you a better physician, nurse, or healthcare worker. For people who are not in the medical profession, this book will help you to take more control of your own healthcare by understanding how to communicate with your physicians and nurses. Regardless of your profession, these communication techniques can prove invaluable in your life. After all, who wouldn't want to learn how to better communicate? Who knows, you may become a better salesman, a better leader, a better partner, the life of a party, or even get that new sports car you always wanted.

For physicians and healthcare workers, "It's all in the delivery" may be the difference between helping or hurting your patients when they need you the most. It may be the difference between having a successful practice or struggling to get referrals. It may even be the difference between healing your patient and a poor outcome. In fact, several studies have shown that poor communication is the leading cause of serious medical errors and the rise in malpractice lawsuits (see Chapter 6).

Improving your ability to communicate effectively and compassionately can save lives, enhance your career, reduce the risk of lawsuits, and make you a better healthcare provider. It is a vital skill that takes guidance, patience, and practice—the same tools that help us to become great physicians, great nurses, great healers.

Chapter 1
How I Got Here

Time has a way of changing our point of view. Yet, certain memories remain indelible in our minds. Visions of distant experiences can seem so clear, as if they happened yesterday. The memories that we can recall immediately shaped the way we see the world today.

For me, there are several vivid childhood memories that help to answer two questions: (1) Why did I want so badly to become a physician, and (2) How did I become so intrigued with compassionate communication? I knew I was destined to practice medicine from the age of 10 or 11. Sure, I may have had the usual fantasies every boy has of becoming a major league pitcher or a professional quarterback, but I always knew I wanted to be a doctor.

I can easily pinpoint the timeline. It began as a five-year-old child spending time in hospitals that I frequented as a boy with epilepsy. Imprinted on my mind is the traffic on the George Washington Bridge as my parents drove into Manhattan from New Jersey every month to see a child neurologist. I remember the grey halls of Columbia Presbyterian Hospital in New York City. I recall sitting in a hard, plastic chair for hours waiting to see the doctor. My recollections of Columbia are not sad or terrible, but what I remember the most, oddly enough, was that everything was grey. The halls, the chairs, the examination room were so gloomy. I hated to go there. It wasn't life threatening or painful, except for the occasional finger prick for a blood test, but mostly I hated the long hours in the car and sitting in a colorless room. The long wait would culminate in the doctor briefly examining me, writing out new prescriptions, and instructing my parents to make another appointment in a month or two. It wasn't good or bad. It was just a part of my life that I accepted.

I suffered from a disease called Petit-Mal or Absence Seizure—a form of epilepsy that causes a child to freeze at any time and stare into space with no response. The word seizure often conjures up visions of people flailing their arms and legs on the ground, biting their tongue, and foaming from the mouth. That is called Tonic Clonic Seizures or Grand-Mal Epilepsy. Fortunately, for me, my particular type of epilepsy is usually controllable with the right medications and is often limited to childhood. Most patients outgrow Petit-Mal by the time they are adolescents. Nevertheless, it can be frightening to a child, and more than 50 years later, having had three children of my own, I now understand how scared my parents were the day I first had an episode.

As with many stories parents often tell, this particular one has become more dramatic as the years have gone by. It was Christmas morning in 1969. There was snow on the ground—how much is unclear. It may have only been two inches, but the amount has increased each time my father tells the story. Just as every father likes to brag about trudging a mile to school through the snow, uphill both ways, in freezing weather, my father took liberties with this story. (As a parent now of nearly three decades, I can more than understand how the trauma of that day would lead to his exaggerated story.)

On this snowy, Christmas Day in Newark, I became unresponsive shortly after opening up Santa's gift. Maybe, at first, my parents thought I didn't like the present. There I stood next to the tree, with my eyes wide open, a blank stare on my face, and not responding to calls, gentle shakes, or light slaps on my face. My arm started to twitch, and panic quickly set in as my very young parents realized something was wrong. My father was a police officer in Newark, N.J., and, as most police officers do naturally, he quickly went into management mode. The emergency person on the phone told my mother that the snow was too deep for the ambulance to get to us. Without any other choice, my father draped me over his back and began walking through the knee-high snow. Or was it waist-high snow? It depends on which version of the story he's telling. The emergency room was about four city blocks away, so wading through the snow was a decent option. As the story goes (and begins to fall apart factually), my grandfather met us in his car about halfway there and took us to the hospital. How his car would make it through the snow but the ambulance could not is a point they tend to gloss over.

Columbus Hospital was a small community hospital in the North Ward of Newark. In the mid to late 1900s, the North

Ward was almost entirely made up of Italian Americans. Like many other immigrants, my great grandparents made their way through Ellis Island to build a new life for themselves. The early years in the U.S. were filled with discrimination and ethnic inequalities. Physicians of Italian American descent were often denied admitting privileges to hospitals. In order to combat this discrimination, hospitals were built to accommodate the many Italian physicians who needed a place to practice medicine. Columbus Hospital was built, and naturally, would be named after one of the most famous Italians, Christopher Columbus.

Columbus Hospital was not strong on academia, but it filled a need for the local Italian-American community. It was mostly run by general practitioners and a few specialists. There was no pediatric ward or, for that matter, a real pediatrician. Therefore, my care was led by my family doctor, Dr. Anthony Merk. Dr. Merk was a typical family practitioner. He did general medicine and pediatrics, as well as obstetrics and gynecology. Born in 1918 as Anthony Mercogliano, he changed his name after suspecting that his ethnic name was the reason he was twice denied acceptance to medical school. Interestingly, after converting his name from Mercogliano to Merk, he was accepted the next year. I would later realize how much Dr. Merk influenced me as a person and a physician. There's a lot more about that later in the book.

Dr. Merk was waiting for my parents in the emergency room when my father arrived. It seemed as if everyone was able to drive in the snow except the ambulance. In any event, Dr. Merk gave me the necessary medications, admitted me for observation, and, as all good general practitioners do, referred me to Columbia Presbyterian Hospital to see one of the best neurologists in the country. And so the memories of the George Washington Bridge and the incredibly grey walls of the child neurology clinic became a familiar site to me for the next eight years.

In between the clinic visits to New York, Dr. Merk would see me in his office and admit me to Columbus Hospital when I had the inevitable breakthrough seizures. I don't have a lot of memories of being in the hospital, but the ones I have remain strong. A few rooms were designated for children, but the nurses cared for all ages on the floor simultaneously. During those eight years, I was admitted perhaps a half a dozen times. With each admission, I hoped for two things: a roommate my age whom I could play with and a bed by the window so I could watch the construction workers use the massive equipment to build the new addition to the hospital.

As with most police officers, my father started out as a beat cop on the night shift, which turned out to be quite advantageous when I was hospitalized. Parents were not allowed to stay past visiting hours in those days, but every night my father, wearing his uniform, would walk past the guards in the hospital and bring me a treat. Suzy Qs were my favorite, I recall weirdly, but Twinkies or homemade cookies were just as good. And my father always brought extra for my roommate. He would sit with me until he got called away by his radio or most often would get chased out by the stern nurses at the desk.

One night, I vividly recall my father acting very much out of character. I had been admitted the night before due to another prolonged seizure. This would happen from time to time and usually only required a tweaking of my medications. That night, I felt especially lucky. It was late and the nurses had not yet shut the television off in my room. I was sitting in bed watching cartoons when I saw my father at the nurse's station in his uniform. He looked mad, yelling and being animated with his hands, demanding that the nurse call Dr. Merk immediately. The nurse, I recall with great detail, replied to his yelling with an explanation that, "It was for his (my) safety because they could not watch me." I hadn't a clue what they were talking about or why my father was so angry. The nurse called Dr. Merk and both she and my very agitated father entered my room. What I didn't know at the time was that I had been placed in what my father referred to as a "strait jacket." After my medical training, I learned that it was more accurately called a posey restraint, which is a harness, usually white, with ties on each end. It is placed around your body with your arms inside and then connected to the hospital bed rails by strings. The purpose is to make sure a patient does not fall out of bed during a seizure. To my father, it was a strait jacket, and even if they called it a posey, his son was tied up and the nurse's inability or unwillingness to watch me was no excuse for tying up his son. At the instructions of Dr.

Merk, the nurse began untying me. As the nurse released me, I was still not quite sure why my father was so upset. The posey had kept me quite warm and cozy in the drafty hospital room. I was happy to see my father but was more concerned that the nurse would realize that she'd forgotten to turn off my television.

As I look back at these events—the colorless hallways of Columbia, the anger my father felt toward the nurses, the late-night calls to Dr. Merk, the painfully long waits in uncomfortable chairs, the deep concern of my parents for their child, my challenges with seizures, and a very caring doctor who "cured" me—I'm sure it all shaped the person I am today and heavily influenced my decision to go into medicine. Little did I know at the time that all of those experiences were the basis of my understanding of the patient experience. Even though time might change our perspective (and definitely alter my father's overdramatic story of that snowy Christmas day), those formative years provided me with the incentive to reinvigorate compassionate communication into the medical profession of today.

Dr. Cunningham

As I enter middle age, I frequently think about how I became so intrigued with communication in healthcare. Perhaps it began as I watched my father yelling at the nurses when I was hospitalized as a kid. Other than that, it's somewhat of a mystery to me. I certainly never imagined I would write a book about it. I guess God has a plan for each of us, and

I believe that His plan for me included teaching compassionate communication to healthcare workers.

As I mentioned earlier, I knew that I wanted to be a doctor from a very early age. The idea of doing something truly significant with my life appealed to me. Also, I was fascinated with how the human body works and how complicated it is. But there was another reason, too. Challenge appeals to me—so much so that I tend to always choose the most difficult challenge presented to me. It is a curse and a blessing at the same time.

I chose medicine because I was told it was impossible to get accepted into medical school. I chose neonatology because it appeared to be the hardest of all the subspecialties. It turns out, one element of neonatology was even harder than I thought—giving bad news. As I entered my fellowship training, the thought of telling someone that their baby died or suffered a catastrophic illness frankly scared me to death. You see, I was blessed. I was 26 years old, had two healthy parents, a wife, and a child on the way. I even had three grandparents who were still alive and well. At that point in my life, I had not yet felt what it was like to experience a real tragedy. That made the thought of telling someone bad news even more terrifying. But it was something I knew was inevitable. Neonatologists deal with life, death, and tragedy every day. There was no way to avoid telling parents bad news.

As a resident in training, I saw senior physicians tell

parents bad news all the time. Some of the doctors seemed to do it well, but some appeared very uncomfortable. Most, like me, were never given any training on how to tell someone they had a life-threatening illness or that a loved one had passed away.

When I give lectures, the most frequent question asked of me is how I came to dedicate so much of my career to teaching healthcare professionals how to communicate with compassion. The truthful answer is that I have no idea. I was just drawn to it, I guess. But there was a pivotal point in my career that I often refer to as the time when I decided this was my passion. (I later learned, as this book will show, there were many more previous events and influences in my life that led up to the development of the communication techniques I now use to teach.)

One incident particularly stands out in my mind. In the summer of 1994, I was a first-year neonatology fellow at Thomas Jefferson University Hospital (TJUH) in Philadelphia. For those of you who may not be well versed on the nomenclature of the confusing hierarchy of medicine, a fellow is a licensed physician who has completed specialty training in a certified residency program but has chosen to continue in their training toward a goal of becoming a subspecialist. In my case, I had the great fortune to have been accepted and completed my pediatric residency program at Thomas Jefferson. To the dismay of my wife, I chose to delay a high-paying job and train an additional three years to be certified to care for the smallest and sickest of newborn babies.

I refer to the six years of training at Thomas Jefferson (three as a pediatric resident and three as a neonatology fellow) as the best professional years of my life. The hospital had a fantastic reputation, and for good reason. They recruited the top people and were a major referral hospital for the region. The neonatologists were, at the time, a who's who in this relatively new subspecialty. The Neonatal Intensive Care Unit in the 1990s was run by Dr. Alan Spitzer. He built a reputation for being a no-nonsense neonatologist who demanded perfection from everyone and created loyalty wherever he went. When Dr. Spitzer came to Thomas Jefferson as the new director of neonatology, he brought with him an all-star team of the smartest, most well published group of neonatologists one would find anywhere. Along with the outstanding neonatologists from Christiana Medical Center in Delaware, I truly believe that it is this group of professionals who contributed to making me the physician I am today. This is not simply because of their amazing knowledge of physiology and medicine, or their intelligence that seemed to be unattainable by me or anyone else. It was much more than the academic knowledge that they shared. Dr. Spitzer and his group taught me that it is possible to be an amazing, gifted physician, with superior intellect and still be a real, down to earth, compassionate person. They truly cared about the residents, fellows, nurses, and staff they worked with and insisted that everyone call them by their first name. In retrospect, they were a major reason that I chose to postpone the six-figure salary of a pediatrician to continue my training for another three years. Their kindness and dedication to the babies and parents were beyond what I had ever seen before. It is for those reasons that this story of the very sick baby that changed my life is even more remarkable and surprising.

I remember the incident as if it were yesterday. It was during the first few weeks of my fellowship training when I received an urgent call from a desperate physician to pick up an extremely sick newborn from a hospital just over the bridge in New Jersey. The baby had Meconium Aspiration Syndrome (MAS) and Severe Pulmonary Hypertension. MAS is a condition that occurs when a newborn baby defecates into the amniotic fluid shortly before birth and then inhales the contaminated fluid into the lungs. The meconium or "newborn stool" clogs up the airways and causes severe inflammation of the lungs. When severe MAS occurs, it can interrupt the normal process of the newborn's heart and blood vessels to adapt to life without a placenta, preventing the major blood vessel leading from the heart to the lungs from opening up enough to allow sufficient blood flow needed to pick up oxygen from the lungs.

This baby had an extreme case of MAS and Pulmonary Hypertension. He had not responded to the aggressive therapy given at the referral hospital, thereby leaving no other option but to emergently transport him to an ECMO center. Extra-Corporeal Membrane Oxygenation, is essentially a heart-lung bypass machine in which a surgeon places catheters into the major blood vessels of the baby's neck. The catheters are connected to a machine that continuously takes the baby's blood out of one catheter, adds oxygen, and returns it back to the baby through the other catheter. It essentially does the work of the baby's lungs until they have had an opportunity to heal.

In the early to late '90s, TJUH was one of the premier ECMO centers in the country, which meant that it would frequently get the sickest of all newborns in the area.

As the fellow in the Neonatal Intensive Care Unit, I was in charge of transports for the month. Since it was early in my training, I was being supervised by the senior neonatologist. Later in training, fellows typically are in charge of NICUs without supervision unless needed. Even though my training at this point was very limited, it was my duty to go in the ambulance with the transport team, pick up the baby, and bring him back to Thomas Jefferson to be placed immediately on ECMO.

Dr. Timothy Cunningham (not his real name), was the senior in charge that night. Famous in his own right, Dr. Cunningham was one of the loyal and gifted neonatologists that followed Dr. Spitzer when he came to TJUH. I had known him for most of my pediatric residency. He was a kind man, an extremely gifted physician, and a true mentor. I looked up to him and wanted to be as good as he was someday. He was a major reason why I chose to stay at TJUH for an extra three years of training for my fellowship.

Tim (he insisted everyone call him by his first name), was soft spoken, dedicated to his work, and showed me how a real physician doesn't leave the bedside when a baby is sick, even if it is time to go home. He also taught me that a true leader doesn't just push everyone to be better. A true leader lifts up everyone around him. The NICU parents and the entire nursing staff loved him. Tim was also the first person to send out a compliment when someone did a great job. He was twice as nice as I thought I would ever be and 10 times smarter than I could imagine becoming. On that night when the desperate call came to pick up the critically ill baby with MAS, I felt very fortunate that Dr. Cunningham was my supervisor.

When I arrived at the hospital in New Jersey, it was apparent that the tension in the room was high. At the referring hospital, the baby was receiving 100% oxygen delivered by a mechanical ventilator that was performing at its limits. I assessed the situation, spoke to the parents, and obtained the necessary consents for transport and placement on ECMO. This was not a procedure to be taken lightly. It is associated with many possible complications, including stroke, bleeding, and infection, but as I explained to the parents, getting their son to TJUH and on the ECMO machine as fast as possible was his only chance of surviving. I politely informed the father that he would not be allowed to accompany his son in the ambulance and got the necessary signatures. The parents gave their son a quick kiss on the cheek and we wheeled the baby as quickly as possible into the ambulance, lights and sirens blasting. By everyone's estimate, there was not much time. The ventilator was failing to keep the blood oxygenation levels up, and despite epinephrine, IV fluid boluses, and every other treatment we had to offer, the baby's heart rate drifted slowly down. I called Dr. Cunningham, who could only add assurance that we were doing everything we could do and that the surgeons were ready to place the baby on ECMO as soon as he arrived. As we made our way back over the Ben Franklin Bridge to Philadelphia, the baby's heart rate continued to drop—the oxygenation of his blood still not adequate.

By the time we arrived, we were performing a full resuscitation including CPR on the baby. Dr. Cunningham took charge of the resuscitation when we arrived. We could not place the baby on ECMO unless we could first get him to respond to the CPR. The surgeons waited, gowned and gloved, to see the outcome of our efforts.

CPR continued and multiple rounds of adrenaline administered but the heart rate never returned. Dr. Cunningham instructed the team to stop CPR and pronounced the baby dead. It wasn't long before the charge nurse informed us that the father had followed the ambulance and was anxiously waiting for an update, completely unaware that his son had died. Dr. Cunningham asked the nurse to have the father wait in his office.

At the time, I saw this tragedy as an opportunity to learn a life lesson. It was a skill I needed to learn desperately but one that scared me to death. A skill that, unfortunately, I would need many times during my chosen career: how to tell a parent that his or her newborn baby passed away. This was a perfect time to learn. After all, who better to learn from than Dr. Cunningham, who was one of the kindest and most intelligent doctors I knew?

I asked Tim if I could come with him to speak to the father and observe how he broke the bad news. Of course, he said it was fine. Without saying another word, we walked together down the hallway to his office that doubled as the on-call room for the neonatologists. We entered the room to find an extremely anxious father pacing back and forth. What happened next was, and still is, inexplicable to me. This gentle and caring doctor, whom I'd come to greatly admire, simply blurted out, "I am Dr. Cunningham. Your baby died."

I was shocked. "Did he just do that?" I thought. The father, who was still standing, was totally blindsided by the news. Total shock set in and the father went crazy. He banged the wall with his fist, screamed loudly, and knocked over the table lamp. I didn't know what to do. He spewed out profanity and screamed in a tone that I had never heard before. Dr. Cunningham froze. He wasn't doing anything. He was just standing there as if he knew he had just done something terribly wrong. I took a step forward and tried to say something to the father, but Dr. Cunningham put the back of his hand in front of my chest and said, "Let him be."

The next minute of screaming seemed like an hour. The father eventually caught his breath and took Tim's invitation to sit down. As the two sat together, I stood in the

How I Got Here   Anthony J. Orsini, D.O.

back, still recovering from the shock of what just happened. Tim seemed to gradually get back to his true character as he spoke softly and with compassion as the father cried. That was the Dr. Cunningham I knew.

After a brief discussion and some more crying, we escorted the father to the room where his dead son lay. We stayed with him for a minute or so and then left him to be alone with his baby. As I walked out of the room, Tim stopped me in the hallway. Standing in front of me, he put both hands on my shoulders and looked me right in the eye. I could see that his tears were swelling. Then, with deep sincerity in his voice, he said in a firm, deliberate, staccato-like manner, "Do you see what I did? Don't ever do that." And without saying another word, he turned and walked away down the hallway toward the fire escape to gather himself, still crying.

That day changed me forever. It affected me profoundly, and increased my already deep fear about communicating bad news. If Tim could mess this up so badly, what chance would I have? This was something I had to learn, and fast. What did he do that made the father react with such anger, or was it just a random reaction? Is there a right way to break bad news, and if so, how can it be learned and taught? The questions swirled in my mind. From that point on, I was determined to learn how to do this. I saw first-hand how, in just a few minutes, the manner in which a physician relays news to a patient or family member can affect them deeply. Doing it right is just as important as any life-sustaining procedure doctors do. But with all the advances in medicine, the medical profession has not seemed to master the simple act of communicating compassionately to our patients and their families.

I finished my three-year fellowship at TJUH and my expectations were fully met. Training with the best made me feel more than prepared to care for the sickest of newborns. There were many more opportunities to observe Dr. Cunningham and the other neonatologists relay painful news to parents. I observed every chance I could. Sometimes the news was horrible, such as a death or a major brain hemorrhage that would likely cause a baby to have severe neurological impairment. Other times, the news was less painful, such as informing a parent their baby would need surgery or had an easily treatable infection. I became more aware that regardless of the severity of the news, the manner in which the news was delivered almost always affected how parents would react in the short-term and cope with the news in the long-term. It would take me years, however, to find the key communication techniques that determined the short- and long-term reactions to bad news.

As I graduated from my fellowship and took my first real paying job as an attending neonatologist at NYU Langone Medical Center, the proper way to deliver bad news still eluded me. After three years of watching the best of the best, three years of reading about the subject, a pattern had still not revealed itself. Time was up, however, and it was my turn to be in charge.

Chapter 2

Compassion in Medicine and How We Lost Our Way

It is well documented that compassion in medicine dimin-ishes as medical students advance through the many years of postgraduate training. Invariably, medical students arrive on the first day of classes, fresh out of college, eager to learn and with a passion for becoming physicians. During the third and fourth years of medical school, clinical rotations begin, and excitement and altruism flow. Fascination with the human body, physiology, and the reality that doctors can actual cure human beings peaks during these years.

After medical school graduation, newly licensed physicians often enter internships at the height of their compassion and are ready to conquer all diseases. The excitement of be-coming a "real doctor" is tempered only by the overwhelm-ing realization that the life or death of a patient is, for the first time, actually in their hands. The stakes are high. One mistake and their career is over, or worse, a patient can die. Dr. Amy Cuddy, a well-known psychologist, discusses in her book *Presence* what psychologists refer to as Imposter Syndrome. Dr. Cuddy defines it as the deep and sometimes paralyzing belief that someone has been given something that he/she didn't earn and doesn't deserve. It occurs when someone worries that they are unprepared for the job that they are doing and constantly worries about what other people think of them.[1] I believe that Imposter Syndrome is universal for all interns and residents.

Although interns and residents are supervised, the responsibilities placed upon them are immense. Residents in training receive the first call from a nurse when a patient has a problem. They are the first line of defense, responsible for ordering appropriate laboratory studies, writing medication orders, and keeping track of every detail about their patients. The hierarchy of medicine dictates that residents and interns examine their patients early in the morning before their seniors arrive and are ready to answer any questions their attending physician or senior resident might ask. Any physician reading this book can readily recall the long hours, sleep deprivation, and immense pressure they were subjected to as residents. I am certainly no exception. The seven years I spent after medical school graduation as a rotating intern, resident in pediatrics, and neonatal fellow were professionally the greatest learning experience of my life. They were also the toughest. Memories of beepers and phones constantly interrupting my thoughts still cause anxiety. Like most physicians, I still don't believe I've caught up on the sleep that I lost more than 25 years ago. Therefore, it's not surprising that the steady stream of demands from nurses, therapists, senior residents, and attending physicians slowly pushes even the most well meaning, compassionate resident into pure survival mode. The excitement of healing patients is slowly replaced with the desire to simply "get through the day or night." Something has to give. This profound fatigue often results in a failure to feel the compassion that was once the impetus for choosing medicine in the first place.

The relationship between this "compassion fatigue" and professional burnout is complex (more on that later). One fact that is indisputable is that both are extremely prevalent among doctors and nurses. For the majority of physicians, compassion peaks in medical school and slowly decreases throughout residency training. Of interest, those who experienced burnout early in their training tended to stay burned out, while those who were not showing signs by the end of their first year generally did not get burned out later.[2-4] Why some physicians suffer from only slight compassion fatigue while others entirely lose sight of why they became doctors in the first place remains a mystery. I believe that it's the people young physicians meet along the way that can, without their knowledge, influence how much compassion fatigue occurs during training. Young physicians are extremely impressionable. Interns observe the behavior of their senior residents and attending physicians like a four-year-old boy mimics his father shaving. Although I witnessed Dr. Cunningham struggle with telling a father his son had died, I knew he was a compassionate person, and over the years, he remained a positive influence on me. His advice to "Don't ever do that" remains engraved deep in my brain. It showed me that he was a genuinely compassionate person even if he did not always know how to communicate that compassion.

Dr. Banks

Several years before Dr. Cunningham gave me that heartfelt warning, I met someone who, at the time, did not seem very important in my life's journey. Years later, however, I would realize that he was a perfect example of what happens when physicians lose all sight of the purpose of why they chose medicine. I graduated from medical school, as most do, with an excitement that I was finally a real doctor but also with the knowledge that I had at least three more years of rigorous days and sleepless nights before I would be ready to have my own practice. Because I hadn't yet chosen a specialty, I decided to complete a one-year rotating internship that would allow me to get another sampling of multiple specialties, much the same way as I did during medical school. I chose Coney Island Hospital in Brooklyn, mostly because it was close to my hometown in New Jersey. It also appealed to me because it was one of the busiest hospitals in the New York/New Jersey area and had a reputation for giving a lot of responsibility to their interns. (This is good for someone who is training, but probably not so good for the patients.) I began my internship in July of 1990, still filled with empathy and excitement.

Shortly after arrival, I realized I had received exactly what I asked for. The place was as busy as Times Square on a Saturday afternoon. The massive emergency room resembled Grand Central Station and had a steady stream of patients flowing in and out 24/7. The huge, newly built emergency room consisted of one very large triage room with a square-shaped, plexiglass enclosed area in the middle, designed for nurses and physicians to write their notes, fill out paperwork, and check lab results on the computer. Around the perimeter were smaller examination rooms.

Down the hallway was the trauma room, the X-ray room, and the plaster room for patients who needed their broken bones casted. Even though the emergency area had just been built, it was already too small to accommodate the large number of patients entering each day.

Patients were registered by the front door and placed on gurneys in the main triage room. The gurneys were lined up in three or four rows of 10 to 12 patients. All with various diseases, they laid side by side for hours, with very little room between them, waiting to be triaged. Once seen by the triage nurse, they would then be placed in a smaller examining room only to wait again for an intern or resident to complete their own examination and decide if their condition was serious enough to require admission to the hospital. Looking back, it was quite surreal and somewhat intoxicating. The fast-paced, mildly controlled chaos resembled a MASH unit in the middle of the Korean war. Things moved fast for the doctors, nurses, and hospital staff, but for the patients who entered the hospital, it was a very different story: wait, wait, and wait. It was not uncommon for a patient to lay in a gurney for more than eight hours waiting to be seen by a physician.

During my orthopedic surgery rotation in December of 1990, I met Dr. Jonathan Banks (not his real name). Jon was a short, athletic-looking senior resident with a hint of Napoleon syndrome. He was 5'6" (at most), walked and talked extremely fast, and treated his patients as if they were broken down cars that needed to be fixed. He did everything fast and took extreme pride in his efficiency—

more specifically, his ability to work the system. Jon was six months away from completing his training in orthopedics. To anyone who was paying attention, he had all the symptoms of a resident whose compassion meter had dipped into the red zone. When I entered medical school, my plan was to become an orthopedic surgeon, but it did not take long after my first few days observing as a student to realize that it wasn't for me. The specialty seemed more like carpentry than medicine. Orthopedic surgeons spend much of their day mixing plaster, drilling into bones, and inserting screws. I believe this carpentry mentality makes it especially easy to forget that the bone at the end of the drill is actually attached to a person. After decades of teaching compassion communication, I consider orthopedic surgeons some of the most difficult students. By mid-year of my rotating internship, I had already decided that pediatrics would be my specialty but, nevertheless, I still needed to complete my rotating internship. For the month of December, that meant getting through orthopedic surgery and working every third night with Dr. Banks.

The first night I was on call with him was memorable. We had just finished hours in the plaster room, splinting and casting multiple arms, legs, and fingers, when Jon headed for the large triage room. As he walked down the hallway in his typical brisk manner, he waved his hand over his head motioning for me to follow. He called out, "Let's go. It's time for hip rounds." I wasn't quite certain what he was referring to, but I obediently followed him down the hallway toward triage. As usual, there were about 30 patients lying on gurneys side by side, in three rows of 10. Without saying a word to me or to the patients, he walked up and down the rows with rapid pace tapping each patient firmly on both of their feet. I watched confused but still followed closely, as all good interns do. What I quickly learned was that he was checking to see if any of the patients in triage might have suffered from a broken hip. When patients break a hip, any rotation of the hip, such as what would occur when someone slapped their feet, would cause extreme pain. When he reached a patient who let out a cry from the pain caused by tapping the foot, he would quickly pull the gurney out of the row, examine the patient, and wheel them down the hall for X-rays. Cutting the line of patients already waiting in the hallway for X-rays, Dr. Banks would position his patient in front of the machine and take the necessary X-rays to confirm his diagnosis. He was almost always correct.

Once the diagnosis was confirmed, Jon would say to me with a proud smile, "I will book her for surgery in the morning. Do the paperwork and get the consent. When the emergency medicine doctor calls you in the middle of the night to admit the patient, tell him that everything is already done and to go back to sleep." Then he'd walk to his call room to get some sleep. He had beat the system.

At the time, I thought the whole thing was quite amusing. How clever, I thought, and now we will both get more sleep. I was in no position to say anything, and quite frankly, didn't think much of it other than I was happy to get a little more rest that night—a commodity that was rare. Looking back, I see Dr. Banks in a very different light. The pain he inflicted on these mostly older patients as he tapped their legs purposely and the manner in which he treated the patient bothers me much more today than it did as a young intern. It wasn't until decades later that I realized Dr. Banks was typical of what happens when you take a young, eager, compassionate medical student and subject him/her to 80-to-100 hour work week and 24-to-36 hour shifts without sleep. They go into survival mode. Some get through it with only minor effects. Others, like Dr. Banks, lose compassion altogether. Understanding this process of compassion fatigue is the first step to avoiding it and returning to the excitement of the young medical student.

The Historic Role of Compassion in Medicine

Believe it or not, compassion used to be the largest part of a physician's job. Prior to the late 19th century, compassion and very rudimentary medical treatments were all that physicians had to offer. The average life expectancy at the turn of the century was only 48 years. It wasn't until 1870 that Louis Pasteur and Robert Koch established the germ theory of medicine, and penicillin was not widely available until the mid-20th century. That amazing, historical fact shows how far medicine has come in a little more than 150 years. Prior to the late 1800s, doctors had little scientific knowledge or medical cures for the diseases they were trying to treat. In most cases, providing comfort was all they could do. Most of us are familiar with early paintings of doctors sitting by a patient's bedside holding their hand while the nurse placed a cold towel on the patient's forehead. Doctors were perceived, and rightly so, as comforters.

They eased the pain as much as possible, with a kind word, some primitive medications, and a lot of compassion.

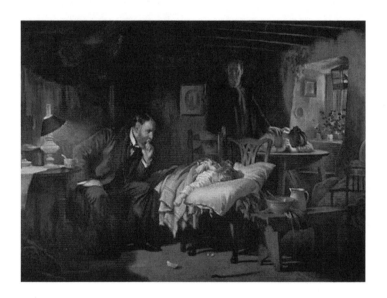

As times changed, medicine became more scientific. Modern medications such as penicillin were discovered and increasingly sophisticated surgical techniques were developed. New procedures and medications were being introduced every day. But as with everything, progress comes with a price. Physicians were holding instruments instead of hands. The human touch was being replaced. Doctors began to see themselves as scientists and healers instead of comforters. The great advances in medicine pulled the human touch away from the doctor-patient relationship to the point where physicians who felt emotions were often thought to be unprofessional or have clouded judgement.

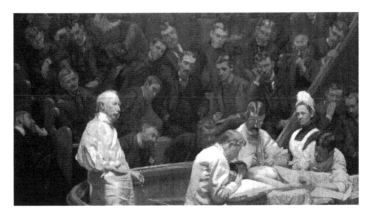

Thomas Eakins. The Agnew Clinic. 1889.

Although this painting dates back to 1889, it represents the changes in physicians' representations beginning in the late 1800s and into the early 1900s.

Medical schools' curricula reflected this new way of thinking. They stopped teaching young men and women how to communicate. Knowledge was emphasized over compassion, and communication skills were rarely mentioned outside of training students to take a patient's medical history. Medical schools became more competitive with their admission criteria and placed an even higher priority on grades rather than the ability of an applicant to be a well-rounded person who could communicate effectively. Schools were graduating a higher percentage of extremely smart individuals who lacked the necessary skills to interact with the average patient on a compassionate level.

This transition is very evident in the famous commencement speech "Aequanimitas" by Dr. William Osler to the graduating class of the University of Pennsylvania School of Medicine in 1889. Dr. Osler is one of the most renowned physicians in history. He was Canadian and one of the founders of the prestigious Johns Hopkins Medical School. He is considered by many as the "father of modern medicine" and is known as one of the greatest diagnosticians in the history of medicine. In his speech to the graduates, which later became an essay, Dr. Osler instructed the class to limit their emotions. He stated, "Only by neutralizing your emotions to the point that you feel nothing in response to suffering, physicians can best see into and hence study the patient's inner life.[5]" In later years, others furthered the instructions and advanced the narrative that doctors should not "feel." The rise and promotion of terms such as "detached concern" (listening empathetically without becoming emotionally involved[6]). and "neutral empathy" (observing a patient's emotions without feeling grief, regret or your own emotions[7]) demonstrates how embedded this way of thinking became in medicine. This new trend, combined with advances in technology, further drove physicians to believe they were more scientists than healers. Compassion became not only a barrier but, as scholars were teaching, a hindrance to good medicine. We lost our way.

As doctors became more scientific and modern medicine advanced, it did so, to some extent, at the expense of compassion, communication skills, and ultimately the ability to build relationships. But the demands of the modern patient have changed and the doctor-patient paradigm has shifted. Until recently, the public fully accepted that one would freely choose a physician with a bad bedside manner if he/

she had a reputation for being an excellent clinician. This is no longer the case. Today's patient also desires a trusting relationship with their healthcare provider. They want to be treated with respect and demand more from their physician than simply just being a good clinician. They seek physicians and nurses who are genuine people they can relate to and who care about them as if they were part of their extended family. Patients accept that every physician has had the proper training and, quite frankly, have no real way of determining which doctor is better than the next. As Fred Lee stated in his book *If Disney Ran Your Hospital*, "Patients assume that their doctors and nurses are competent just as we all assume that the pilot flying our plane knows how to fly.[8]" Patients choose their hospitals and physicians by referrals from friends and stay loyal only if they feel a strong relationship with their healthcare provider. The pendulum has swung freely since the days of Dr. William Osler and is now pointing in the other direction. If hospitals and physicians are to be successful both financially and clinically, their doctors, nurses, and team members must be able to build lasting, trusting relationships with their patients and families. The "good doctor with the lousy bedside manner" has gone away.

Compassionate Communication in Medicine

Compassionate communication is the ability to share ideas and feelings both effectively and with compassion. It is how we use our verbal and non-verbal skills to communicate not only information to patients and families, but to convey a true commitment to ease their pain. Only when patients genuinely feel compassion can they truly trust that their healthcare provider has their best interests at heart.

Compassion and empathy are related but are not the same. The term compassion literally means "to suffer with." It is defined as the feeling that arises when you are confronted with another's suffering and feel motivated to relieve that suffering. In order to feel true compassion, you must use your imagination to place yourself in the patient's situation. It is the only way to truly feel and, therefore, connect. Empathy comes much easier and is defined as the "understanding of one's pain or situation." Understanding and feeling are two very separate things. Empathy can be faked, but true compassion must be felt, and that requires imagination. To paraphrase the 17th century philosopher René Descartes, "I feel, therefore I am."

Empathy + Imagination = Compassion

Over the years, I have had the privilege of working with many professional actors. As we will discuss later in this book, the Breaking Bad News program I developed to teach communication uses professional actors who portray patients while doctors practice delivering tragic news to them. It is fascinating to watch the actors get into character just before the scene starts. They accomplish this by imagining what it would be like to have just lost a child or been told they have cancer. Actors know that using their imagination is the only way to truly play the scene. It is not enough to simply pretend to be the patient. The actors have to "become" the patient. The same concepts apply to medical professionals when having a difficult discussion with patients. It is easy for us to get caught up in the rapid pace of the day and become task-oriented. We can forget that we're about to change a patient's life forever, and to them, we are the most important person in the room. Before any meaningful conversations can take place, you must take a moment and place yourself in the patient's shoes. Stop to take a breath and imagine. This is half the battle. By doing this, your non-verbal language will be consistent with your words and the patient will genuinely feel a connection with you.

Doctors and Communication

Why is effective and compassionate communication such a challenge? What can we learn from the history of medicine about how physicians have traditionally thought about compassion, feelings, and communicating with their patients and their families?

Let's face it, communication has never been known to be a strong suit for physicians. We are all familiar with the stereotype of the brilliant but nerdy doctor who has limited social skills. Of course, this characterization does not fit every doctor. There are many well-rounded physicians who are excellent at building rapport and interacting with their patients. However, as with most stereotypes, they are born from common traits consistently present over many generations.

When you consider what it takes to pursue a career in medicine, it is easy to see why this label has some validity. Being admitted to a medical school in the United States is extremely competitive; only applicants at the top of their class get accepted. Traditionally, medical schools base their admission on grade point average (GPA) and the medical college admission test (MCAT). Very little is based on the applicant's life experiences, past successes, or even his/her ability to communicate. Yet, we are somehow surprised when our doctor is unable to communicate effectively, or even worse, unable to form a relationship. Nurses, on the other hand, are generally better at communicating and forming trusting relationships with their patients. They tend to be more equipped from the onset. By the nature of their job, they are "people persons," and because they spend a considerably longer amount of time at the patient's bedside, they have more opportunities to bond and get to know their patients. The time they spend with patients administering medication or making sure their bed is in a comfortable position or even helping someone with the television in the hospital room gives them a greater opportunity to have casual conversations, which leads to deeper bonding. But even with more opportunities for meaningful interactions, evidence shows that nurses, as a whole, also struggle with compassionate communication.

In recent years, some medical schools have started to place more emphasis on the applicant's real-life experiences as well as their ability to communicate and succeed in the real world. But ideas come easy, and implementing change happens gradually, so this new approach has been slow to catch on. Some admissions departments that have traditionally boasted about the average GPA of their applicants, compared to those of other medical schools, have met this idea with some resistance.

The healthcare industry spends billions researching best practices, finding new medications, and inventing new procedures. Physicians take courses to improve their skills and earn Continuing Medical Education credits. Hospitals pay large sums of money to become certified by JCAHO (Joint Commission on Accreditation of Healthcare Organizations) or to be MAGNET® designated for nursing excellence in order to show that they are safe and practice good medicine. Risk management departments spend their days with hospital attorneys to improve consent forms and create policies and guidelines. Many of these well-intentioned and necessary policies only make medicine less personal and further drive a wedge between the patient and the healthcare provider.

To be honest, it has always baffled me that hospitals will readily pay large amounts of money to improve safety or be designated by a third party as "better," but are reluctant to spend any money teaching doctors, nurses, and staff how to communicate. Communication techniques, especially when handling bad news, is the "third rail of medicine." In other words, something no one wants to talk about. The healthcare industry has chosen to ignore this as a factor for a number of reasons:

- Communication and compassion are difficult to measure

- Communication techniques can be diffiult to teach

- It is uncomfortable to talk about and no one wants to be told they are not good at it

- It is not considered important enough to spend time teaching it

Being able to communicate effectively and with compassion is half the battle in helping patients get well. Yet, studies have shown that during a patient/physician interview, the physician interrupts a patient an average of every 11 seconds[9]. In the most basic terms, physicians who are unable to listen, or who try to multitask while the patient is speaking, can miss important facts about the patient's complaints or symptoms. From the patient's point of view, these clinicians will be perceived as disconnected and uncaring, impeding any relationship with their patient. Without a trusting relationship, patients will be less likely to follow the treatment plan and, therefore, more likely to experience less than optimal outcomes.

There are several references to studies pointing toward the importance of effective and compassionate communication in medicine[10]. Patients who believe that their doctor feels genuine compassion for their situation and has communicated well with them are more likely to:

- Take their medication

- Follow prescribed treatments

- Experience better outcomes

- Rate their physician or hospital higher
  on patient satisfaction surveys

- Not file a malpractice lawsuit even when
  a mistake has been made

Relationships based on compassionate communication are part of the bedrock of good medicine.

How Doctors Think

In the well-known book *How Doctors Think*, Dr. Jerome Groopman tells the story of a young woman, Anne Dodge.[11] For more than 15 years, Anne had suffered from severe abdominal cramping, diarrhea, and vomiting. Despite eating more than 3,000 calories per day, her weight had fallen to just 82 pounds from malnutrition. Her bones had become so weak they resembled the bones of an 80-year-old woman. She had already seen dozens of doctors and received various opinions from multiple specialists, including psychiatrists, all of whom were unsuccessful in making a diagnosis. As a last attempt, and with pressure from her family and friends to see just one more doctor, Anne finally agreed to see Dr. Myron Falchuk.

By the time Anne came to Dr. Falchuk's office, she was

extremely weak and nearly suicidal. Doctors didn't believe that she was eating the prescribed calories and had labeled her illness as psychological. She visited Dr. Falchuk, believing the outcome would be exactly the same— he would dismiss her symptoms, prescribe more meds, and send her home. To her surprise, however, the doctor took a very different approach. He did not look at the thick chart sitting on his desk. Nor did he read the test results from the multitude of studies other physicians had ordered. Instead, he just sat with her and listened. At first, Anne was reluctant to speak. After all, her past experiences led her to believe that nothing would change. But this doctor was different, she thought. He asked her open-ended questions, affirmed her feelings and concerns with his non-verbal language, and encouraged her to continue speaking. Anne believed that Dr. Falchuk really cared, and a trusting relationship formed quickly. She felt more and more motivated to share her symptoms and her emotions. Anne finally allowed Dr. Falchuk to perform further tests, which eventually led to the diagnosis of Celiac Disease. At that time, Celiac Disease was thought to be quite rare, especially in adults. With more sophisticated testing, we now know that it is much more common than previously thought. The disorder did not allow Anne to digest foods properly and metabolize nutrients from food, no matter how much she ate. Dr. Falchuk's ability to communicate with Anne and convey true compassion allowed Anne to trust him in just one visit. The mutual respect they had built in just a short time was the first step toward the correct diagnosis and subsequent treatment. At the instruction of Dr. Falchuk, Anne changed her diet and her symptoms slowly resolved. At her one-month follow-up visit, she had gained more than 12 pounds and her symptoms were all but gone.

In modern medicine, patients are no more than vessels for a group of symptoms, and their diagnoses are riddles that need to be solved. Patients are often referred to by their disease: the diabetic in room 302, or the kidney failure in room 375. Physicians are trained to approach patients with a series of algorithms. Does the patient have this? If yes, go to the next line. If no, proceed to the next question. At a superficial level, it seems like a very efficient way to think. Unfortunately, it requires no communication skills and strips the human interaction between physician and patient down to a quick physical and a prescription. The story of Anne Dodge emphasizes the need for physicians to master the art of communicating effectively. Without relationships, the doctor-patient interaction is no more than a series of imperfect computer algorithms.

It's All in the Relationship

As discussed earlier, the late 19th and early 20th century brought new technologies to the field of medicine, transforming physicians from healers to scientists. Toward the end of the 20th century, two related events occurred almost simultaneously, further burying compassion beneath layers of responsibilities. First, insurance companies lowered their reimbursement amounts, forcing doctors to see more patients in less time. Second, the rise of HMOs put a priority on the number of patients seen rather than the outcomes or the quality of care. Physicians, feeling more and more rushed, looked for new ways to be efficient. Nurses and physicians became increasingly more task-oriented rather than patient-oriented. This new arrangement caused patients to feel more like numbers than people. Sitting in a waiting room or emergency triage for hours only to be seen by a doctor who examined them quickly and asked questions while typing notes on an electronic device made medicine very impersonal. Something was missing. Patients wanted to be treated with respect. They wanted a relationship with their doctor.

To paraphrase Sir Isaac Newton, "With every action there is an equal and opposite reaction." Unintended consequences occur with every change. Predictably, patients unhappy with the impersonal feel of medicine began to complain about their care, and the rising popularity of the internet gave them a new, very public forum to express their opinions about the care they received. Patients were given the opportunity to rate their doctors online and review their experience during hospital and office visits. Patient satisfaction surveys such as HCAHPs (Hospital Consumer Assessment of Healthcare Providers and Systems) were developed by the government to assess hospitals and physicians.

Two worlds were colliding. How could physicians and nurses be expected to see patients at a record speed, write extensive notes to avoid lawsuits or denial of payments, and still establish the one-to-one connection that patients demanded? The answer breaks down to one simple word: relationships.

Forming relationships is difficult to do in a short period of time, but it can be done. Yet, the deck is stacked against physicians learning how to do this well, starting with medical school admission requirements that traditionally did not consider real life experiences or the ability to communicate. Add to that the minimal allotted time spent with patients, lack of training, and lack of role models, and it is not surprising that the same applicants are now physicians who have difficulty forming relationships with their patients. The good news is that communication skills can be taught. Healthcare providers who understand the proper verbal and non-verbal techniques of communication can learn to form trusting relationships with their patients in a short period of time. In the following chapters, I will outline the simple, yet vital, steps necessary to communicate well, build trusting relationships quickly, and produce healthier, happier patients.

Chapter 3

The Special Case of Breaking Bad News

Although this book is about communication in medicine and how it affects every aspect of healthcare, the task of breaking bad news is perhaps the most difficult of all types of conversations. It has been my experience that healthcare providers who can deliver tragic news effectively and with compassion are frequently the most skilled at communicating with their patients under all circumstances. However, the fact remains that very few physicians feel comfortable giving bad news to patients, and most healthcare providers report that the mere act of breaking bad news results in personal anxiety and stress. Most physicians cite two reasons for their associated anxiety: lack of training and fear of getting it wrong. For the most part, physicians understand the impact difficult conversations have on their patients, and while they want to help, they simply have not learned the proper methods of delivering bad news.

Why is it so important that these difficult conversations be done the right way? The manner in which someone receives bad news can affect them not only in the short term but for decades that follow. Patients and families can readily recall even the smallest detail about the moment that their lives changed forever. The clothes the physician was wearing, the proximity of which everyone was seated, and even the color of the walls can frequently be recalled decades later.

I still remember the unique, shrieking tone of my mother's scream early one morning when she heard from a nurse on the phone that my grandfather had died. I can remember the exact spot I was standing as a young, 14-year-old getting ready for school and the position on the bed that I found my mother sitting when I ran upstairs to console her. The tragic news that a patient or family hears can, quite literally, change their lives forever. At the exact moment they hear the news, they are transformed from a healthy person to someone with cancer, from a parent to someone who has just lost a child, or from a husband or wife to widow or widower. The words they hear from the physician and the manner in which they hear them can either help or hurt when they are at their most vulnerable. That is a tremendous responsibility for anyone. Add lack of proper training and it easily explains why these types of conversations are viewed as a dreaded task instead of a skill to be proud to have mastered.

In truth, doctors are considered by many to be especially poor at breaking bad news. In a retrospective study by Finlay and Dallimore entitled *Your Child is Dead*, parents who had experienced the sudden death of their child were asked to rate the attitude of the person who delivered the news. Physicians' delivery of the news was twice as likely to be rated as "offensive" or badly handled" than police officers.[12] As a whole, physicians give bad news far more often than police officers and nurses, yet are much more likely to be considered unempathetic. The notion that repetition breeds improvement is clearly misleading. To use a sports analogy, swinging a baseball bat the wrong way 1,000 times per day will result in a player who is very skilled at swinging a bat incorrectly. Repetition only results in improvement when proper instruction is given in the first place. If physicians are going to break the stigma of being cold and uncaring, they must receive compassionate communication training early in their career and have good role models to emulate as they practice this important skill.

Although medical schools are slowly introducing communication training into their curriculum, it is still lacking, and the vast majority of physicians and nurses remain untrained. Those who have been trained either received short, didactic lectures or learned by watching senior physicians who may or may not have been good communicators themselves. It has always baffled me that something that affects patients and families so profoundly and can cause such anxiety to healthcare professionals would not be emphasized more during medical school and residency programs. Without proper training and good role models it is logical that having difficult conversations is such a source of anxiety. This was certainly the case for me.

Teaching, learning, and practicing compassionate communication, especially in the special case of breaking bad news, is about changing the culture. It is about bringing the topic of compassionate communication to the forefront of all conversations. Senior physicians must place a higher priority on teaching communication skills to medical students and residents. Early in their career, residents need to be given the proper skills and knowledge to have difficult conversations and be encouraged to pass those skills to the next generation. Communication skills, especially as they relate to handling difficult conversations, must be redefined not as a task but a skill of which to be proud. Every aspect of medicine except for communication training has the same procedure for teaching: learn about it, watch it, assist someone doing it, do one with assistance, and finally, do it yourself. When it comes to learning how to break bad news or communicate properly, the procedure is much simpler: learn about it briefly, followed by go ahead and do it. Most would agree that it would be unsafe and, frankly, absurd to provide a one-hour lecture on performing appendectomies and then send someone into the operating room suite to perform one on a real patient. Yet that is what we do when teaching compassionate communication. It takes time to learn appropriate communication skills and must be treated with the same importance as an appendectomy or any other major procedure done by physicians.

For instance, during daily hospital rounds, it is customary for attending physicians to ask the medical students and residents questions to assess their knowledge and teach important aspects of the care of each patient. Communication, however, is rarely discussed on daily rounds. Occasionally, residents will be asked if they have contacted the family to give updates, but accepting a simple "yes" or "no" reinforces communication as a task to be checked off on a "to do" list. Instead, senior physicians should ask the resident about the specifics of what was said during the conversation and how it was delivered. Personally, I have placed a high priority on communication skills during resident rounds. Invariably, the first time I ask young residents and practitioners to elaborate on the quality of the conversation and specifically how they communicated with parents, I often receive confused and almost annoyed looks. Their facial expression speaks loudly: "What do you mean what did I say?" Repeating this line of questioning with the residents every day on rounds reinforces the message that proper communication is an important skill that must be learned. After a few days, residents and students quickly come to understand the point of the "how did you communicate" questions. The message is heard loud and clear. It is not enough to just speak to the patient. It is what you say and the manner in which you say it that really counts. By teaching young physicians how to communicate early on in their careers, they will feel more confident about their skills, feel less anxiety during the difficult conversations, form better relationships with their patients, and, most importantly, help their patients and families when they are most vulnerable.

By placing communication skills as a priority, it becomes just as valued as any diagnostic skill. Each are important and depends on the other. As Dr. Groopman explained through the story of Anne Dodge, great communication skills are required of any outstanding diagnostician. We can sometimes learn from those who possess the skills and use them often. Yet, impressionable healthcare workers without the proper base-knowledge must make sure they are "swinging the bat" properly. Palliative care providers are especially good at having difficult conversations. The wise physician or nurse can learn from watching those skilled at communicating. But, sadly, examples of poor communication among doctors and nurses are more prevalent, and without proper training, the ability to discern the good and the bad can be difficult. Teaching these skills early allows physicians and nurses the opportunity to complete continuing education courses that reinforce those skills throughout their careers. Having difficult conversations in medicine is a lifelong learning process. I'm still learning after all these years. I still learn from patients and families. I suspect I will never stop.

My First Time Breaking Bad News

Several years after Dr. Cunningham walked toward the fire escape with tears in his eyes, I had still not made much progress learning how to discuss bad news. It wasn't for lack of trying. There simply was not enough information or enough role models from which to learn. In 1997, I finally had my first real job. At the completion of my training, I was fortunate enough to land a job at New York University as a full-time neonatologist. NYU Langone Medical Center had a Level III NICU in a teaching hospital. I was confident that my training at TJUH prepared me well, and I started with confidence that I could not only survive but add some qualities to the already excellent group of neonatologists. My new boss, Dr. Karen Hendricks-Muñoz, was very much like the neonatologists at TJUH. She was very supportive and quick to compliment but demanded excellence. In a world where intelligence is common but quality leadership is rare, Dr. Hendricks-Muñoz had both.

As a new attending neonatologist acclimating to my new environment, Dr. Hendricks-Muñoz gave me limited clinical responsibilities to allow my confidence to grow. I started in July, and by September, I found myself solely responsible for the care of approximately 50, very sick neonates. During that first month as an attending, Dr. Hendricks-Muñoz checked up on me without being judgmental, and with each visit, her words of encouragement reaffirmed me. As each day passed, her nods of approval combined with the confidence that my training at TJUH was top notch, helped convince me that I belonged at such a prestigious hospital. Throughout the month, I was caring for twin baby girls who were barely two months old and had been in the NICU since they were born at just 25 weeks gestation. They had a difficult course with ups and downs and suffered many of the complications that often occur when babies are born 15 weeks early. Several times that month they became critically ill, and each time, I used my resources and training to pull them through. One complication common in premature infants is called Retinopathy of Prematurity or ROP. This is a disease that occurs when the blood vessels of the retina grow abnormally and is usually a result of being born early and requiring large amounts of oxygen. Mild cases of ROP are of little consequence, but in rare cases, the blood vessels grow so abnormally that there is a risk of retinal detachment and blindness. The good news is that if the severe ROP is caught in time, blindness can often be prevented with treatment.

As the neonatologist in charge, it was my job to tell the parents that one of their daughters would need laser surgery to hopefully prevent blindness from her severe ROP. The procedure is usually successful but, despite aggressive therapy, blindness or limited sight is still a possibility. This would be my first time giving bad news without the safety net of someone else in charge. Having seen first-hand how delivering bad news incorrectly can affect parents, I was naturally anxious. I took this very seriously and arranged for a family meeting with the parents in the nearby conference room. This is often done in neonatology to update parents, but mostly when the conversation requires a multidisciplinary approach. Trying to recall the few lessons that I learned from observing difficult conversations with parents over the past six years, I did my best to speak softly and kindly and told the parents that if their daughter was to avoid blindness she would need laser eye surgery right away. Phew, I thought. It was over. I did it. But it was not over. The mother of the twins let out a shrill scream that resembled the one I heard from my own mother when my grandfather died. She fell off her chair and sat against the wall. Still screaming, she started to repeatedly bang the back of her head against the wall over and over again, screaming toward heaven, "Why? Why?" I thought, Oh my God, I had learned nothing. It's Dr. Cunningham all over again. I put my hand between her head and the wall to prevent her from hurting herself but pulled it away when the pain from my crushed finger told me it wasn't such a good idea. It was my first attempt as a neonatologist giving bad news and I blew it. I hadn't learned anything. My next thought was that I needed to learn how to do this and I needed to learn fast, both for my patients and for myself. All the confidence I had built over the past month had just dwindled to nothing. Sure, I could run a code blue or treat the most critically ill infants, but when it came to helping families when they needed me the most, I was still clueless.

I was more determined than ever to find the answers to two very important questions that had plagued me for years. Is there a right way and a wrong way to deliver bad news to a patient or family? And, if there is a right way, how can it be taught?

For the next 10 years, I dedicated myself to finding the answers. I continued to watch as many physicians as possible. I read what little literature there was on the topic. I admittedly learned through trial and error, but most importantly, I interviewed dozens and dozens of family members and patients who were very willing to share their experiences with me. It was through these interviews that I learned the most about what patients and families need and how to help when they need it the most.

The History of Breaking Bad News

In 2000, Walter F. Baile and his colleagues published a manuscript introducing a six-step strategy for delivering bad news using the acronym SPIKES (Setting, Perception, Invitation, Knowledge, Emotion, Strategy) (see Table 1, pg. 71). Over 500 attendees of the 1998 Annual Meeting of the American Society of Clinical Oncology (ASCO) were asked a series of questions to assess attendees' attitudes and practices regarding the delivery of bad news. The study found that although more than 98% of clinicians polled reported delivering bad news at least five times per month, less than 12% rated their ability as very good. Most reported as being "not very comfortable" when asked about their ability to handle their patient's emotions. This prompted the need to introduce guidelines based on consensus for clinicians to discuss bad news, and the SPIKES protocol was introduced. SPIKES provided much needed instructions for physicians on how to discuss life-altering topics with patients and families.[13] Although SPIKES was a groundbreaking effort to supply some guidance for physicians, I believe, through the years of my personal research, that several of the concepts no longer apply to the modern patient. SPIKES places a large emphasis on providing information. This was certainly appropriate when the program was published almost 20 years ago. However, with new, universal access to the internet, today's patient has instant availability to information, thereby shifting the goals of effective and compassionate communication less toward providing information and more toward relationship building. In addition, SPIKES was developed specifically to aid physicians when delivering tragic news and not intended to be used as a guide for routine interactions between patient and healthcare provider. Although some of the concepts of SPIKES have become less pertinent to the modern patient, it still remains the most commonly taught method in medical schools. Yet in my experience teaching communication, few residents and senior physicians can recall the concepts.

Goals of Disclosing Bad News — SPIKES

1.   Gathering information

2.   Transmitting the medical information

3.   Providing support to the patient

4.   Developing a strategy or treatment
       plan with the patient

In order to meet the needs of the more modern patient and provide guidance to healthcare providers on proper techniques for effective and compassionate communication that would apply for any interaction, I developed the BBN P.R.O.G.R.A.M.® acronym (Plan/Position, Review, Observe, Gradual/Genuine, Relationship, Accountability, Meet) (see Table 1). I believe this method of care has two distinct advantages over the SPIKES method. First, the concepts apply to all types of interactions including routine conversations as well as more difficult discussions such as delivering bad news. Second, the BBN P.R.O.G.R.A.M acronym places emphasis on relationship building whereas SPIKES is directed more toward providing information.

Communication Rule #1: Don't be a Google doc. It's not just about information!

During decades of teaching, I have found that, by far, the most common mistake made when delivering tragic news is the belief that the goal is to provide as much information to the patient as possible. This is the result of the failure of traditional teaching to keep up with the more modern patient combined with the increasingly more litigious nature of medicine. Lawyers and insurance companies view healthcare not as a human interaction but rather a legal transaction that must be protected with full disclosure. Providers feel immense pressure to include every medical detail about the serious condition they reveal to their patient. Accurate information is certainly necessary for patients to make informed decisions and to understand the diagnosis and prognosis. Too much information, however, especially after the initial shock of hearing bad news, is not helpful and will often result in more confusion. It is extremely important that any information necessary for the patient to process must be given before the final diagnosis. Once patients hear the diagnosis, they retain only a small amount of the information that follows. The initial reaction is shock, and the mind begins to process the life-changing words that they just heard. They essentially become incapable of listening. So, say what you need to say first, before giving the bad news. Then, take a breath and pause. There will be opportunities to discuss the details about the disease later when the patient has had time to digest that initial conversation and is more capable of understanding. Remember that the moment a diagnosis is delivered, the patient's or family's life will change forever. Give them time to absorb this new reality.

Three Goals of Breaking Bad News

The goal of any difficult dialogue is not to deliver as much information as possible. If done correctly, the patient and family leave the conversation feeling three important things:

1.   The patient and family should believe that
      their physician understands their situation
      and is genuinely compassionate.

2.   The patient and family should believe that
      their physician is the expert in the room
      and trust that they will lead them to the
      next step. Patients should feel as if they
      are able to put their arms around the
      physician and he/she will guide them.

3.   The patient and family should believe that
      their physician will not abandon them.

The physician or nurse who understands that giving bad
news is less about information and more about connecting
on a human basis will best serve their patients and families
when they are at their most vulnerable.[14]

Teaching Communication

More than a decade of research, trial and error, and numerous interviews led me to the development of the BBN P.R.O.G.R.A.M. acronym as a mnemonic device for the essential components of compassionate communication. Through years of determination, I finally concluded that there really is a right way and a wrong way to break bad news—and it is about a lot more than just being nice. What still eluded me was how to best teach what I had discovered to other physicians and practitioners. This, perhaps, was the harder of the two objectives I had identified so many years earlier. Communication has traditionally been a very difficult skill to teach, especially when it involves pure, raw emotion. Many insisted that being a good communicator is nothing more than a personality trait and could not be taught. I was told by my peers that the ability to communicate is innate: you either have it or you don't. I found the opposite to be true. After training thousands of doctors, nurses, and other medical providers, I can say with certainty that almost anyone can learn to communicate with compassion provided it is taught using the proper format. Simply put, communication skills can't be learned by listening to a lecture or webinar. Communication must be taught the same way as any other important medical skill or difficult procedure: through practicing. Didactic lectures are of very limited use when teaching communication. They provide a cursory introduction to basic concepts, but without immediate application, the lessons are quickly forgotten. Expecting a student to master the advanced techniques necessary to navigate difficult conversations simply by listening to a lecture is almost impossible.

I have found that interactive workshops that encourage class participation are slightly more effective and provide the best option for large groups. As with any difficult skill, however, mastery takes practice.

"Tell me and I forget.
Show me and I remember.
Involve me and I understand."

The best way to learn the art of communication is through experiential learning. However, not just any type of experiential learning is appropriate. I certainly found that out the hard way. Through the years, I have tried various teaching models ranging from peer-to-peer role playing to using volunteers as simulated patients. Although some of these models were slightly more effective than simple lectures, teaching healthcare professionals how to communicate serious news requires more than conventional role playing. It requires improvisational role playing that must be realistic and authentic so as to touch the emotions of those participating so real learning can take place.

Table 1 — Comparison of SPIKES and BBN P.R.O.G.R.A.M.®

SPIKES	
S –Setting: "Setting up the interview." Shut off phones and beepers. Find a quiet spot.	**K–Knowledge:** "Giving knowledge and infor- mation to the patient." Warn the patient that bad news is coming. "Unfortunately, I have bad news."
P–Perception: "Assessing the patient's percep- tion." What have you been told about your medical situation so far? What is your understand- ing of why we got the MRI?	**E–Emotion:** "Addressing the patient's emo- tions with empathic responses." Observe the emotions of the patients. Name the emotion.
I–Invitation: "Obtaining the patient's invitation." How would you like me to give you the information about the test results? Would you like me to give you all the information or sketch out the results and spend more time discussing the treatment plan?	**S–Strategy and Summary:** Discuss a treatment plan, but first ask the patient if they are ready for such a discussion.

BBN P.R.O.G.R.A.M.®

P–Plan/Position:

Have a good plan before starting. Imagine. Think about how you want to deliver the news. Position everyone in the room in the appropriate spot. SIT DOWN. Be ready to change the plan if necessary.

G–Gradual:

Lead up to the bad news gradually. SHOW, DON'T TELL. Don't prepare them for the bad news by saying you have bad news. Use your body language and review to show them that you have bad news. "I am glad you brought your wife in to discuss the biopsy." Telling someone you have bad news IS the bad news.

R–Review:

Review the events that are leading up to the tragic news. Be the attorney. State your case first. Get on the same page. Ask about their understanding of the situation.

R–Relationship:

The most important goal of any interaction. Use relationship words such as "I" and "the." Silence is a powerful message that you care.

O–Observe:

Observe how the patient and family react to the news. You may have to rephrase the information if their reaction is not what you expected. Pay close attention to your own body language. It's absolutely necessary that your verbal and non-verbal language is consistent. Show compassion. Use silence when appropriate.

A–Accountability:

Let them know that you will not leave them. "I will help you get through this."

M–Meet:

Let them know the next step. The patient should not leave your office without a clear understanding of the next step and timeframe.

The Winding Road to Success — Bob Lukasik

After years of attempting to train medical students and residents how to break bad news to patients and families, I was becoming increasingly frustrated with my failed attempts to teach what I had learned. My research led me to the key components of compassionate communication, but I had not yet found an effective model to teach young physicians how to properly convey difficult news to patients. My first attempt used peer-to-peer role playing: asking one resident to play the role of the patient while the other delivered the news. The amateur acting and the familiarity of the residents with each other resulted in little more than giggles and embarrassing moments for everyone involved. The scenes were not life-like and, except for bringing some attention to the subject, this teaching model fell short of what I hoped to accomplish. My second attempt used volunteers from the hospital as actors. Some were teenagers who needed to fulfill their community service hours for college and others were parents and family members of patients who donated their free time to give back to the local hospital. Again, the acting was poor and the scenes unrealistic. The results were not much better. Around this time, I heard about the increasing popularity among medical schools of using simulated patients to teach medical students various skills ranging from doing a proper history to performing physical exams. Therefore, my third attempt was to use simulated patients to play the roles of patients and families. Although this model was a big improvement from the volunteers, many of the simulated patients still lacked the depth of acting skills necessary for the more emotional scenes. I was failing miserably.

In 2010, I was fortunate enough to meet Bob Lukasik and Cheryl Galante. Bob and Cheryl ran a local production company in New Jersey that produced several plays per year for a popular neighborhood theatre. When we met, I discussed the failed attempts at finding an authentic and effective teaching model to train young physicians how to deliver bad news to patients and families. Bob listened carefully and then told me the story of how he was informed of his mother's death more than 15 years earlier. He had arrived at the hospital to visit his mother and asked the nurse where he could find her. The nurse pointed to a room and said, "She is in there. She's dead." Bob's voice cracked while telling the story as if he had still not recovered from the nurse's harsh words. I had hit a nerve with Bob and he immediately jumped at my suggestion to use his professional actors to portray patients and family members in the scenes. I pointed out that there were limited funds available to pay actors of that caliber. With tears in his eyes, he answered, "We will make it happen."

The skills of professional actors would solve two problems identified from the past failed models. First, real actors allowed us to make the scenes improvisational. It is important to allow actors to have the freedom to react to whatever emotion they are feeling during the scene. That is the whole point of the training: to teach the participant that the reaction from the patient is not random but rather a response to how the news was delivered. For instance, if the physician's verbal or non-verbal language is perceived by the actors as uncaring, the actors might feel anger and react accordingly. If the physician spoke with compassion, the actors would react very differently. In my experience, only professionally trained actors can truly do improv. In addition, in order for the physician to really experience the raw emotion that often occurs during the most difficult conversations, the scenes must be realistic. Even with cameras in the room, the skills of the actors immediately immerse the physicians into the scene and they often forget that the actor is not a real patient.

Even with Bob's assurance to "make it happen," there was still cost involved and administrators in the graduate medical education departments who were reluctant to devote the time and money to what was often called a "luxury." In 2010, I approached Dr. Mary Ann LoFrumento, who was the assistant pediatric residency director at Goryeb Children's Hospital and long-time leader at Atlantic Health, and explained my frustration with getting the program approved. What is most impressive about Mary Ann is her no-nonsense, get-it-done attitude. She has never had patience for politics when medicine or teaching is concerned. Dr. LoFrumento listened to me as I explained my program and objectives. Her response was the final piece of the puzzle I needed. "Let's just do it and ask permission later," she said. So, in January of 2011, the first Breaking Bad News program was offered to 36 pediatric residents at Goryeb Children's Hospital in Morristown, New Jersey.

The residents were given two scenes, each with a task to complete. The scenes required the physicians to break bad news, ranging from telling parents that their five-year-old child suffered a severe brain injury from a near drowning to informing a mother and father that their nine-year-old had died suddenly from septic shock. To enhance the teaching experience even more, I recruited non-medical instructors, most of which had lost children or have heard physicians deliver terrible news about their own children. The non-medical instructors would add feedback from a layman's point of view, as well as add credibility to the lessons taught by the medical instructors. The sessions were videotaped live and reviewed with the physician immediately after the scene had ended.

From the first scene, I knew we had hit upon something special. The raw emotion from the professional actors and their ability to improvise what they were feeling from the doctor delivering the news made it real. Many of the residents left the room crying as they looked at Dr. LoFrumento and me with tears in their eyes, saying, "That was so real, and I didn't know what to say," as Mary Ann gave them the hug they were seeking. That is exactly the point, I thought. This could have been a real patient or family they were speaking to, and because they were not properly trained, they would have had no idea what to do to help. Similar to the realization that I had come to after the mother of the twins fell to the floor and banged her head against the wall almost 20 years earlier, the young doctors suddenly understood that the art of breaking bad news was a skill they must master...quickly.

The review of the videotaped scenes was equally emotional. I used the BBN P.R.O.G.R.A.M.® acronym (discussed in more detail later in this chapter) as a roadmap to help the resident physicians understand the key components of effective communication. After their quite dramatic realization of how important the skill of breaking bad news was, each physician hung on every word of advice from the instructors in the review room. Instructors pointed out the subtleties of body language as well as the tone, cadence, and inflection of the words they spoke when giving the news to the actors. The video component was crucial to the teaching, allowing the participants to see the nuances of the messages they were trying to deliver. It's one thing to tell someone that their non-verbal language was too casual or the pace of their speech too fast. It is quite another to show someone on video.

The results were nothing less than life-changing for everyone in that room but especially for me. The feeling I had that day will never be forgotten. I knew at that moment that I had finally accomplished what I had set out to do nearly 20 years earlier.

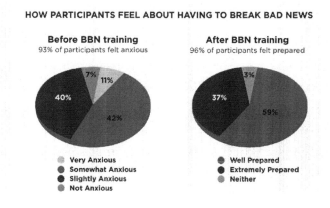

HOW PARTICIPANTS FEEL ABOUT HAVING TO BREAK BAD NEWS

Before BBN training
93% of participants felt anxious

7% 11%
40%
42%

● Very Anxious
● Somewhat Anxious
● Slightly Anxious
● Not Anxious

After BBN training
96% of participants felt prepared

3%
37%
59%

● Well Prepared
● Extremely Prepared
● Neither

Later that month, I gave a presentation to the entire hospital, showing excerpts from the videotaped scenes as well as the results on the effectiveness of the unique program. The local news picked up the story and the rest is history. I have been teaching communication skills ever since. I am proud to report that since 2010, the Breaking Bad News® program has individually trained more than a thousand residents, senior physicians, nurses, and even first responders in almost every medical specialty around the United States. This doesn't include the thousands of others who have attended introductory lectures and workshops. Sadly, Bob Lukasik died in 2019. However, his determined statement, "We will make it happen," has rung true. Cheryl Galante and the actors and actresses at the production company remain a vital part of my communication training.

Essentials of Communication Training

- Scenes must be improvisational. Do not give actors a script.

- Use professional actors who are skilled at improvisation.

- Scenes should be realistic.

- Videotape scene while instructors watch in a remote room.

- Use medical and non-medical instructors.

- Review scene immediately after role-playing session.

- Review must be positive and constructive. Participant must feel comfortable.

The BBN P.R.O.G.R.A.M.® — A Roadmap for Compassionate Communication

With the exception of SPIKES, which was introduced in 2000, little or no guidance has been provided on how to communicate with patients and families. The BBN P.R.O.G.R.A.M.[14] is a guide on how to communicate with patients and families during difficult conversations and helps to build trusting relationships during routine encounters. It is not meant to be memorized and regurgitated in robotic fashion. Instead, it is to be used as a roadmap for teaching effective communication techniques and concepts. These techniques can also be used as a springboard into establishing a relationship with patients and families, and the mnemonic device of the title makes it easy to remember.

If you haven't figured it out already, BBN stands for Breaking Bad News. To review, the P.R.O.G.R.A.M. acronym means: Plan/Position, Review, Observe, Gradual/ Genuine, Relationship, Accountability, Meet. As we go through this chapter, I will explain each step of this vital process in detail.

To be clear, I believe that the majority of healthcare professionals I have encountered during my career are compassionate individuals by nature. Although this compassion may be natural, conveying it is often difficult. Medical providers often cite time constraints and self-preservation— fear of the overwhelming emotion involved with giving news that is the cause of so much emotional pain—as a reason they have not mastered these skills.

The first step to becoming proficient at any task is learning how to do it correctly. It is natural that physicians and nurses feel anxious about having tough conversations. Few were taught the proper way to navigate difficult discussions. This prompted the need for an effective teaching tool as patient-centric medicine evolves. The concepts of the BBN P.R.O.G.R.A.M. are equally effective, whether telling someone about the death of a loved one or in any situation in which you need to really connect with another individual.

P–PLAN/POSITION

It always astounds me how many people enter any important conversation—whether they are giving tragic news, speaking to an angry patient, attempting conflict resolution, or even trying to make a sale—without a plan.

Before entering the room, you must know what you want to accomplish and how to get there. Planning is the foundation for all meaningful conversations. Yet, many healthcare professionals mistakenly assume that time constraints do not allow them the luxury of sitting down and having a meaningful conversation with their patients. In fact, having a well thought out plan will actually save time. Anticipating the patient's reaction and delivering the news correctly will likely avoid disbelief, distrust, and the questions that follow. As Mark Twain once said, "If you want me to speak for three hours, I'll start right now. But, if you want me to speak for three minutes, I need a week to prepare." Even if it's only one or two minutes, take that time to come up with a plan.

Of course, there is always the possibility that the family will not react the way you anticipated, so be ready to change the plan if necessary.

Regardless of whether the news is a broken leg or a sudden death, the first step of any plan is to imagine. Every sound plan starts with your imagination. Imagine what it would be like to hear the news from the patient's perspective, then make your plan. Keep in mind the three goals of delivering bad news:

That the patient and family believe:

1.   **That you understand their situation and are genuinely compassionate.**

2.   **That you're the expert in the room and will lead them to the next step.**

3.   **That you will not abandon them.**

Remember that your beliefs and opinions of what is important may be very different than your patient's, so it's imperative to put yourself in their shoes. Ask yourself how devastating the news will be to the patient's family. Bad news comes in all shapes and sizes. To one person, bad news may simply be being told they will not be able to participate in the championship basketball game due to a knee injury. To others, it may be hearing they have cancer or a loved one has died unexpectedly. Clearly missing an important game and having terminal cancer are not equally life-changing diagnoses. However, we must remember that to the patient, both are terrible news. Patients and family members don't perceive the news as a choice between missing a basketball game or dying of cancer. To them, both are devastating and, therefore, both should be treated with the utmost of care. If you imagine what it would be like to be the patient, you will be ahead of the curve and ready to formulate a good plan.

Case Study — Thomas McMaster

I first met Thomas McMaster and his family when I was a fourth-year medical student doing my clinical rotation in pediatric cardiology. Thomas was a 16-year-old from a small town just outside of Pittsburgh. His father drove a truck and his mother taught preschool. By all accounts, Thomas had a bright future. He excelled in every sport, but basketball was his real passion. By the time Thomas was a junior in high school, he was captain of the basketball team and had Division 1 scouts at every game. He was on top of the world.

His father's dream was to send his son to college. Yet, even with two jobs and picking up extra hours driving, he knew it was unlikely he would be able to afford the high tuition without a scholarship. Fortunately, Thomas has several colleges offering him full scholarships to play basketball. Life was working out perfectly.

I was a medical student working with Dr. Hemant Patel when Thomas and his family came to his office. Three weeks earlier, Thomas had fainted during routine basketball drills. He quickly gained consciousness and the coach told his parents that it was most likely due to dehydration. As was common for Thomas, he had come to practice early that day to do extra drills before the rest of the team arrived. Everyone assumed that Thomas was just pushing himself too hard. After the first incident, Thomas agreed to take it easy for a few days and returned to play in the next game putting on quite an impressive show for the college scouts in the stands. Several days later, Thomas experienced another syncopal episode (fainting) at practice. This time, the coach insisted that Thomas get medical clearance before the next game. His pediatrician sent him to Dr. Patel who was the local cardiologist in the small town.

The family arrived on a Wednesday morning. Thomas insisted that the appointment be made in the morning so he could get back to school in time for his 3:00 p.m. practice. He even came dressed in his basketball practice clothes ready to dart out of the office to do drills. Dr. Patel and his staff did the routine testing for any athlete with syncope. This included a thorough physical examination, EKG, and echocardiogram. Even before testing was completed, I knew that Dr. Patel had already suspected Thomas might be suffering from a condition called hypertrophic cardiomyopathy. Any fourth-year medical student would know that it is at the top of any differential diagnosis of an athlete with fainting spells. For a non-clinician reading this book, hypertrophic cardiomyopathy is a thickening of the heart muscles, especially the pumping chambers called ventricles. In most cases, this is not a life-threatening disorder, and with proper medications, patients can live a long and normal life. Unfortunately, people with this disorder are at risk for sudden death during exertion. For Thomas, this meant that his basketball career would come to a sudden halt. He would no longer be able to play any sport that had the potential to increase his heart rate.

Shortly after the testing confirmed our diagnosis, Dr. Patel asked Thomas and his parents to meet him in his office to go over the results. Thomas asked how much longer he would be held captive because practice would be starting in just a few hours.

Dr. Patel's office was rather large with a desk facing the door and two chairs on the opposite side. Immediately to the right, closer to the door, was a small couch. As Dr. Patel began to speak, Thomas sat on the couch, with basketball in hand, while his parents sat in the chairs listening to Dr. Patel delivering the news.

Dr. Patel said with a sense of relief on his face. "The good news is that the diagnosis was made early, and with the proper treatment, Thomas will live a normal life."

Coming from a family that placed a high priority on sports and being a high school athlete myself, I remember thinking it was odd that Dr. Patel would phrase this as "good news." Thomas' father replied, "Okay, that's great doctor. We have a good insurance plan, so just give us a prescription so he can get back to practice. He has a big game tomorrow and scouts from Penn State will be there."

Dr. Patel looked confused. "I don't think you understand. Any strenuous activity, even with medication, could cause sudden death. Thomas will not be able to play sports anymore." He continued without a pause, "But, thankfully, we caught it early, so he should be okay." Dr. Patel still seemed bewildered by the parents' faces. I knew that he clearly didn't understand how absolutely life-changing this news was to Thomas and his family. Thomas, who had barely been paying attention, picked his head up and said firmly, "I am fine. This is crazy. I am going to practice."

Thomas' life was centered around sports. It was his identity. This was not the news he expected, and predictably, a natural reaction of defiance and total denial followed. The news was equally devastating to his father. His identity was also changing. For years, he had enjoyed his own celebrity as the father of a future Division 1 basketball player. He was quite used to hearing people sing praises about his son. Now, instead of praise, he would hear condolences. Understandably, his dad also received the news with defiance and denial. His mom, on the other hand, reacted to the news quite differently, feeling guilty that she had not taken him to the doctor after he fainted the first time. After quite a short conversation, his father stood up, politely thanked Dr. Patel, and informed him that they would be seeking another opinion. They left while his mother cried.

Although surprising to Dr. Patel, the reaction from Thomas

and his family was quite predictable to me. Some of my fondest memories are being on the high school football field while my entire family was in the stands. Similar to Thomas' family, sports were a way of life. As a high school athlete, I would have considered missing one game as a devastating thing, let alone being told my sports career was over. To Dr. Patel, basketball was just a hobby to be enjoyed and, therefore, it was difficult for him to understand that to Thomas and his family, sports were their identity and their ticket to an education.

It is essential for healthcare professionals to remember that not everyone has the same life experiences. What is important to one person may not be important to another. Dr. Patel failed to imagine what it would be like to be Thomas and did not have an appropriate plan when he entered the room. To Dr. Patel, he was delivering news of relief: that the diagnosis was caught early. Framing the diagnosis of hypertrophic cardiomyopathy as anything but devastating caused Thomas and his father to react with anger, denial, and distrust toward Dr. Patel. Remembering the three goals of Breaking Bad News, Dr. Patel failed the first goal: Thomas and his parents did not feel genuine compassion from their doctor. This is not to suggest that Dr. Patel wasn't compassionate. He simply failed to convey that compassion because he did not identify the needs of the patient.

Whenever planning an important conversation, think of yourself as if you were directing a movie. Before starting a scene, a good director places the actors at a precise spot on the set. Looking back at the case study, Dr. Patel should have had Thomas and his parents sitting on the couch together. Thomas being in the background only added to the disconnect, making it more fantasy than reality to him.

Communication Rule #2: Never ask a question unless both answers are acceptable.

Vital to every plan is positioning, so position yourself for success. It is extremely important that everyone be comfortably seated before any critical conversation takes place. It sends the non-verbal message that you, as the one delivering the news, are not in a hurry, and that you understand the seriousness of the situation, and it is the first step toward meeting all three goals of delivering bad news.

As the expert in the room, you know that it is never acceptable for your patient to receive the news standing up. It's not enough to simply ask the patient and the family if they would like to sit down. Instead, pull out a chair and instruct the patient and family to sit. If there are multiple family members present, move the chairs to where you would like them to be. If the patient or family states they would feel more comfortable standing, tell them that you would be more comfortable if they sat. Pull out a chair, hold your hand out, and gesture toward the chair. Then wait, and wait some more if necessary, until they all are seated. The non-verbal message is that the conversation will not begin until everyone sits down. If there are not enough chairs in the room, go and get them from the hallway. This will further send the message that this is an important conversation. In

The Special Case of BBN   Anthony J. Orsini, D.O.

25 years, I have never had a patient refuse to sit down using this method. Another rule to remember is never sit down until everyone else in the room has already taken a seat. Once you sit down, it will be very difficult to get others to follow. Finally, don't start to speak until everyone is seated.

Chairs Move

As important as it is to have everyone sit before having a conversation, it is equally important to arrange the chairs where you would like the family to be seated. Remember, you are the director of the scene. This is most likely the first time they have heard such serious news, so positioning everyone where you feel is most appropriate is part of any good plan. After years of teaching communication and the art of breaking bad news, I remain perplexed at how many clinicians will sit across the room when having a difficult conversation because "that's where the chairs were." Here is a very important tip: chairs move. Arranging them appropriately for the delicate conversation helps with another integral part of breaking the news: do it gradually. (This will be discussed in more detail later in this chapter.)

Ideally, chairs should be positioned so that you can make eye contact with everyone in the room and close enough to touch (e.g. a comforting hand on the shoulder), if appropriate. If the conversation is with more than one person, arrange the chairs in a triangle or semi-circle so that you can make eye contact with each person. A common mistake is sitting between a patient and his/her family members.

This results in the awkward "ping pong" head, as it becomes necessary to look at multiple family members as you speak. If possible, avoid giving tragic news from behind a desk or table. Furniture is not only a physical barrier, but also an emotional one.

Key points to a good PLAN

- Imagine what it would be like to be the patient or family hearing the news.

- Sit down. Position everyone in the room properly. You are the director.

- Anticipate the reaction you will receive and be ready to adjust your plan if the reaction is different than expected.

- Remember the three goals of delivering bad news.

R—REVIEW

The first "R" in P.R.O.G.R.A.M. stands for Review. An appropriate review accomplishes two very important things. First, it allows the patient and the clinician to get on the same page. There may be, for instance, a minor detail about the history that the physician gets wrong. If that happens, he/she will instantly lose credibility. In addition, patients and loved ones may later feel, no matter how unrealistic, that if they had just had the opportunity to tell the doctor one more piece of information, the outcome would have been different. The time spent getting on the same page also allows for observation on both sides. While the patient is speaking, the clinician is interpreting the patient's and the family's non-verbal cues. The clinician's non-verbal cues are also being observed simultaneously by the patient. The second and most important reason for the Review is that it paves the way for the bracing moment before the patient hears the tragic news. A good rule of thumb is that a proper review should end with the patient anticipating that the news is coming before it is heard. Remember, you are dealing with people during an extremely irrational and emotional time. A good review will help brace them for what they are about to hear.

Here are some guidelines for a proper review. I generally suggest that you start by saying, "Tell me your understanding of what is going on." Let the patient speak and watch their body language. If it is news such as a sudden death, do not let the review go on too long. It may be necessary to guide the conversation a bit by filling in the gaps while they are speaking. The process will not end well if you let the family speak for an extended period of time giving every detail and then tell them their loved one has died. On the other hand, a diagnosis of cancer or a non-fatal disease would allow for a longer review by the patient and family. REMEMBER — If there is no review, it will almost always lead to disbelief and anger.

State the Evidence First

Before stating the diagnosis or giving tragic news, it's very important to make your case first. Build up to the news gradually, giving the evidence first and then the diagnosis. I have taken some tips from my attorney friends who tell me the proper way they are taught in law school to give a closing argument to a jury. Lawyers generally are not taught to say, "The defendant is guilty, and let me tell you why." It is more effective to tell the jury, "Here is the evidence, and this is why he is guilty." The same holds true when giving a serious diagnosis. Telling someone that they have cancer first, followed by an explanation of how the diagnosis was made just adds to the confusion and doubt. After hearing bad news, very few facts are heard and even fewer are retained. Remember goal number two: patients should believe their healthcare professional is the expert in the room. Experts always state the evidence first and then reveal their diagnosis.

As with the attorney's closing argument, a proper review adds credibility to the result. A patient needs to understand how you as the clinician came to the diagnosis. In order to begin the trusting relationship, the patient and family must believe that this conclusion was made only after careful consideration and that the physician also shares in the burden of pain. The review serves as an opportunity to lead up to the tragic news gradually and avoid blindsiding the patient. A well-done review will prepare them for that reality. Therefore, they should expect the tragic news before it is even said.

Communication Rule #3: Give the diagnosis in lay terms first.

Doctors and nurses are taught to speak at an elementary school level. We are told to use lay terms as much as possible when describing a disease, a procedure, or a test. Yet today, we live in the internet era where every word or phrase is easily googled. Trust is not a given for today's patient. They want to do their own research. It's likely that the moment a patient gets home, they will Google what they have heard. To do this, it is necessary for them to remember the diagnosis and how to spell it. The next time you tell a patient a diagnosis or procedure name, watch their reaction. A glassy look appears on their face as their eyes roll up just slightly. What they are doing is attempting to remember the word and how it is spelled, not paying attention to the description in lay terms that follows. In contrast, when patients are given the lay description of the diagnosis or procedure first, they will retain what they have heard. Patients will still desire to look up the term later, so follow your explanation with "we call that," and more importantly, "I will write it down for you before you leave." This allows the patient and family the ability to listen to everything you're explaining and still use Google when they get home.

In our BBN courses, we often roleplay and give examples of both how to do a good review and how not to do a review. The following is one of those exercises.

Example of a poor review: Christopher Peterman was a 52-year-old construction worker, loving husband, and father of four boys. He was driving home from work when he was involved in a motor vehicle accident. He hit his head and suffered a broken left leg. A routine CT of the head was performed shortly after arrival and his leg was splinted.

The CT scan showed no evidence of hemorrhage or trauma. However, to the surprise of the emergency medicine physician, a moderate to large tumor was noted. When the physician entered the patient's room, Christopher and his wife waited anxiously to find out if he could be discharged. Upon questioning, Christopher informed Dr. Jones that he didn't remember what happened during the crash, which only supported the doctor's suspicion: that Christopher's brain tumor caused him to have a seizure resulting in the crash.

Dr. Jones tells Christopher that the CT scan of the head showed a large tumor in his brain. He explains a likely scenario is that the tumor caused a seizure while driving and that is why he does not remember the details of the crash. Christopher and his wife react very differently than the physician expected. Christopher laughs nervously and asks the doctor if he has the right patient. "I got into a car accident. I am not a cancer patient," Christopher says with a nervous laugh. Since Christopher and his wife did not hear any evidence leading up to the diagnosis, it is no surprise that their reaction was disbelief.

In the preceding example, Christopher's response was that the doctor must have had the wrong patient. As mentioned earlier, it's well accepted that patients and families will retain only about 10% of what is said after hearing the tragic news. Dr. Jones did not take the time to connect the dots from explaining how a car accident ended up with a diagnosis of a brain tumor. Because Christopher's doctor did not state his case first, he lost all credibility. Christopher and his wife lost all trust in his competency.

What could Dr. Jones have done that would have resulted in a very different response? First, he should have prepared Christopher and his wife for the bad news by using non-verbal and verbal cues. Sitting down, for instance, next to Christopher's bed and telling his wife that it is good that she is present, would indicate that it is going to be a serious conversation. Next, Dr. Jones should have formed a plan by taking a moment and imagining that Christopher and his wife believed this was a routine car accident that resulted in a simple fracture of his leg. The plan should always include a proper review designed to bring the patient and their family along the path of the physician's reasoning.

Here's a much better way to handle this tricky situation.

Dr. Jones first tells Christopher that he has the results of his CT scan. After thanking Christopher's wife for being there, Dr. Jones begins by saying, "I am going to bring up a chair so I can sit with you. I believe you told me that you didn't remember how the accident happened. Is that correct?" Christopher answers, "Yes." The doctor asks: Have you had any other recent incidents when you couldn't remember things accurately? Any headaches? Any forgetfulness? If he answers yes, then he is building his case and preparing them for the unexpected news. Even if Christopher says no, the doctor is still setting up the following conversation.

"As you know, your leg is broken and we will get that taken care of as soon as possible, but first, I want to go over the results of the CT scan of your head with you. As I mentioned when you came in, it is pretty routine to get a CT of the head when someone is in a car accident, especially if the patient doesn't remember what happened. The main reason for the CT is to look for any trauma or bleeding, but sometimes, even if there is no bleeding, we find something we did not expect. (PAUSE) I just reviewed your scan with the radiologist and he confirmed that there is a mass in your brain. (PAUSE) I believe this mass or tumor most likely caused you to have a seizure and lose control of the car. I am sorry." (PAUSE)

In the second example, the EM physician took the time to bring Christopher and his wife along his path of reasoning. He explained why the CT of the head was obtained and prepared them for the news by sitting down and telling Christopher that sometimes there are unexpected findings on the CT. By stating that he reviewed the CT of the head with the radiologist and then presenting the evidence before the diagnosis, he was able to prepare Christopher and his wife for the unexpected news and send the message that the diagnosis was only made with reluctance and deep thought. Don't underestimate the impact of the pause. Pauses allow for processing and underline the importance of what was just said. In this example, Christopher and his wife are more likely to react to the terrible news with sadness instead of disbelief. Stating the evidence first allowed Dr. Jones to establish himself as a caring, compassionate physician who reviewed the evidence carefully, consulted with the radiologist, and made the diagnosis as the expert in the room.

Always make your case first. Tell your patients the reasons why you are concerned, why you obtained the studies you did, and how you determined that they have a particular disease, cancer, and what were the circumstances that happened to the patient that led up to his or her death.

Note: Some have suggested that the doctors should ask the patient how he/she would like to hear the news. In other words, is the patient the type of person who wants details or to be given the news abruptly? With no prior experience and not having the knowledge of the best way patients cope with bad news, it is an impossible question to answer. What if the patient said, "Just give me the bottom line doctor." Should the clinician blurt the news out that they have terminal cancer while everyone is standing? Of course not. That would end up with similar results that Dr. Cunningham received.

O—OBSERVE

As medical professionals, we are all trained observers. We were taught early on in medical and nursing school to observe the patient, observe the family, and observe their interactions. Is the patient in pain? What are the family dynamics? Most would agree that physicians and nurses are pretty good at observing their patients, but we do not always remember that we are being observed as well. This is especially true during difficult dialogues.

Communication Rule #4: If verbal and non-verbal language are not consistent, it will almost always result in anger, confusion, and distrust.

Every second, the human brain makes millions of assessments on body language. Within less than a second of meeting someone, the ancient brain has determined if someone is a threat or a friend. Therefore, make sure your body language is consistent with the message that you are delivering. Remember, 70% of all communication is non-verbal. When a patient or family is waiting for a diagnosis, they will likely be nervous about the news they are about to hear. From the minute you walk into the room, they are making assessments about your body language. They are looking at your face and watching the way you sit down. They are trying to decide whether this is going to be good news or bad news. The human brain cannot understand two conflicting thoughts at the same time. For example, one cannot be told that it is dark outside and light outside at the same time. Given that information, the brain must decide what is true. The same holds true when verbal and non-verbal language are not consistent with each other. For instance, telling a patient that you are deeply sorry for the loss of a loved one while you are standing up or sitting casually in a chair sends conflicting thoughts (see Picture 1). Your verbal language says, "I am compassionate," while your non-verbal language says "this is a casual conversation and I don't really understand the life-changing effect." Since our brains cannot understand two conflicting thoughts and 70% of language is non-verbal, patients will almost always choose the non-verbal signal they are receiving: the doctor is not compassionate. Therefore, it's essential to every plan that both verbal and non-verbal language send a consistent message designed to achieve all three goals of delivering tragic news.

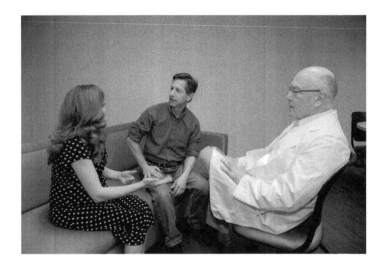

Picture 1:
Example of casual body language. Although the physician took the time to position his chair in an appropriate manner, he is sitting in a very casual manner with his legs crossed, leaning back in the chair. This may be suitable during a conflict resolution scenario such as having a discussion with an unhappy patient. Using this posture and body language while telling someone they have cancer or a loved one has died, no matter how compassionate his voice or words might be, conveys to the patient that the doctor is taking this diagnosis very casually.

The Importance of Silence

"Before one speaks, ask yourself if your words would improve the silence." – Hasidic Rabbi

The proper use of silence is one of the most powerful, non-verbal techniques we can use to connect with another person and show real compassion. Whether breaking bad news to a patient or attempting to resolve conflict with an unhappy patient or employee, sitting silently and listening is crucial to the emotional message you want to send. Without saying a word, silence tells the other person that you are comfortable with the situation, that you are not in a hurry to leave, and you genuinely want to help. Unfortunately, silence is not an easy skill to master. When people feel anxious or uncomfortable, it is a natural response to want to retreat to a safe space. For physicians, our safe space is the classroom or morning rounds. During training, we spend years regurgitating medical facts to our professors and mentors. This is what is most familiar to us and makes us feel most at ease. It is logical that physicians who feel uncomfortable about a conversation would react to a patient crying by spewing out medical terms and explanations of the disease process, even though we know the patient is in no position to listen. It is important to understand that avoiding silence is a defense mechanism for ourselves and does not help the patient or their family. To be skilled at handling any difficult conversation, one must be comfortable with silence. When I get nervous during a difficult conversation and find myself speaking too much, I remember the wise words of Dr. Rabbi Kushner: "Say you're sorry, and then shut up."[15]

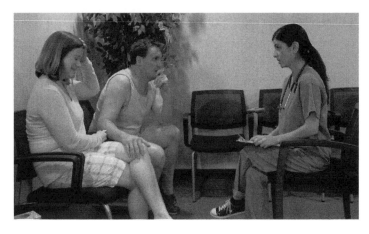

Picture 2:
Here's an example of what I call "Let's keep this professional." Although this physician put herself in a nice little triangle, having the chart on her lap and being so far away from this family places an emotional barrier between them as opposed to the example in Picture 3 that says, "I care."

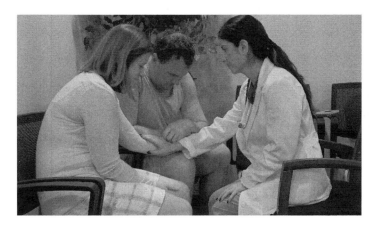

Picture 3:
As I often say during my seminars, I should be able to take any pictures outside to the hallway, show them to somebody and say, what kind of conversation is occurring here? This shows an example of caring and compassion. Even without the touch of the arm, the close positioning and forward lean of this physician shows compassion. It is very important to always be aware of your body language.

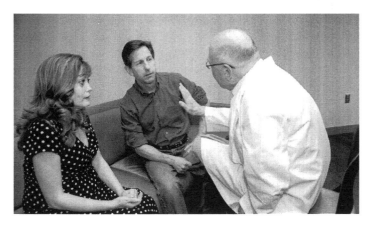

Picture 4:
Don't do this when a patient or family member is upset. Despite our best efforts, sometimes a patient or family member will react with anger, especially if they feel something has not gone smoothly (see Chapter 7, Conflict Resolution). Placing your palm up will only escalate the situation. Instead, reach over with your palm down. It will calm everyone down.

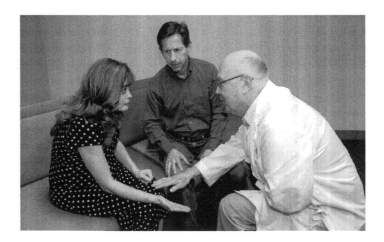

Picture 5:
Difficult conversations sometimes result in anger or disagreement. Reaching out with your palm down and speaking in a soft voice is a good technique to de-escalate the situation. It also redirects attention to the physician and the topic at hand.

G—GRADUAL or Genuine

This, in my opinion, is the most important element of breaking bad news. During routine interactions, the G is for Genuine, but that will be covered in a later chapter. For a more difficult or serious diagnosis, the G stands for Gradual.

Always, always, always break bad news gradually. Never blindside patients or family members. Never give them the diagnosis right away, even if they ask you to do it quickly. As we discussed, healthcare providers feel real anxiety when having difficult conversations. Due to lack of training, Breaking Bad News is naturally viewed as a task instead of a skill of which to be proud. And like most tasks, humans want to complete unwanted tasks as soon as possible. This will result in the common mistake that Dr. Cunningham made many years ago. I cannot emphasize how important preparing someone for bad news is to both short and long-term coping mechanisms. So even if someone says, "Doc, give it to me straight," the proper response should be, "Well, let's sit down first and I promise I will tell you everything you want to know." Remember that you are the professional who has been trained and, therefore, know that it's best to first prepare the patient and family properly by sitting them down, positioning yourself properly, and doing a proper review.

Communication Rule #5: Telling someone you have bad news is not preparing them for the bad news at all. It IS the bad news.

Gradually does not mean drawing the eventual news out.

Properly done, one can actually break bad news gradually in less than a minute or so, but it is extremely important to build to that bracing moment—that moment right before you give the news. The SPIKES technique for discussing bad news teaches physicians to give a warning shot in order to prepare them for the bad news. But giving a warning shot is really not an effective way to prepare the patient and family for what they are about to hear. *Telling an anxious patient that you have bad news is not preparing them for the news at all. It IS the bad news and will result in instant panic and anxiety.*

Communication Rule #6: Show, don't tell.

When preparing a patient for bad news, it is best to refer to the literary rule of "Show, don't tell." Movies and books only occasionally tell the viewer the year that the story takes place. For example, instead of showing *1956* on screen, the director uses cars and clothes from that era. The same is true for delivering terrible news. In the second example of Christopher Peterman, Dr. Jones stated that he was glad Christopher's wife was present and then he sat down. The underlying message, even if subconsciously interpreted, is that it will be a serious conversation. Disseminating less critical news such as a simple broken leg would not need a support person to be present.

By utilizing a proper plan, appropriate review, and consistent body language, a healthcare professional can allow for the all-important bracing moment. Following is an example of delivering news gradually.

The Ambulance Scenario

John Thompsan was a 65-year-old male who began to experience chest pain while mowing the grass on a hot summer afternoon. He called out to his wife, Lorraine, who promptly called 911. The paramedics quickly confirmed John's suspicion that he was having a heart attack and immediately transported him to the hospital. John was speaking as he entered the ambulance and told his wife not to worry because he would be fine. Lorraine called their adult son, who picked up his mother and drove to the hospital to meet John and speak with the doctors. In the ambulance, John began to experience worsening chest pain and shortness of breath. His breathing became irregular and the paramedics were forced to intubate him and start assisted breaths on 100% oxygen. Despite their best efforts, John's status continued to deteriorate and his heart rate began to slow. As the ambulance arrived at the hospital, the paramedics were performing CPR. The Code Blue continued in the emergency room, but despite aggressive resuscitation, Mr. Thompsan was pronounced dead before his wife and son could arrive. John's wife and family were asked to be seated in a private waiting room for the doctor to speak with them.

Bad Technique:

"Ms. Thompsan. I am Dr. Hernandez." Lorraine and her son jumped to their feet. "Doctor, how is my father? How is he?" Dr. Hernandez answered, "I am afraid I have bad news. We did everything we could, but I am afraid we could not

save him. Your father died a few minutes ago. I am sorry."
Lorraine let out an angry scream and said in an accusatory
manner, "That's impossible. He was speaking to me when
he got into the ambulance. He said he was fine. What did
you do to him? What happened?"

In this example, Dr. Hernandez did not use a proper
review and/or have an appropriate plan. He was influenced
by John's son who demanded the news right away and,
therefore, he did not allow for the all-important bracing
moment. Lorraine and her son were blindsided. Not understanding how John could have gone from speaking to his
wife to death in such a short period of time, they reacted
with anger and disbelief.

How should Dr. Hernandez have better prepared Lorraine
and her son for the bad news?

Good Technique:

"Ms. Thompsan, I am Dr. Hernandez." Lorraine and her
son jumped to their feet. "Doctor, how is my father? How is
he?" Dr. Hernandez replied, "I will tell you everything, but
please let's sit down first. My understanding is that your
husband was conscious and speaking when he was placed
in the ambulance. Is that correct?" Lorraine replied, "Yes."
The doctor continued, "While he was in the ambulance,
his chest pain worsened and his breathing became irregular. The paramedics had to put a tube into his airway to
help him breath. Despite giving him medication and 100%
oxygen, his heart rate continued to drop. When he arrived

here, the paramedics had just started CPR (Pause). My team and I continued to do CPR and, despite all of the medications, we could not get his heart to start again. I am so sorry but your husband and father has died."

In the second example, Dr. Hernandez did not give in to the son's demand for immediate information. By having them sit down (Position) and doing a proper Review by telling them the events that led up to John's death, Dr. Hernandez better prepared them for the news. The news is still devastating, but instead of anger and disbelief, their reaction would more likely be met with extreme sadness. In the second example, it is likely that both Lorraine and her son knew that Dr. Hernandez was going to tell them John had died before his last sentence.

R—RELATIONSHIP

The second "R" in P.R.O.G.R.A.M stands for Relationship. Relationships are the key element of healthcare and the goal of all communication.

The age of the internet has changed the needs and demands of the modern patient. When I teach compassionate communication, I often ask the participants what their primary objective is when speaking to a patient or family member, especially when delivering bad news. The most frequent answer I get is, "To provide the patient with the most accurate information." My follow-up question is, "If that is your objective, why don't you just hand him a Google doc and leave the room?"

Of course, my sarcastic response is designed to make a point. As physicians, our goal is not to simply provide information. It's to form a relationship with that patient and family. As I mentioned earlier, patients need to believe that there is an expert in the room who genuinely cares about their situation and will carry them through the next steps.

One might be surprised at how simple changes in a word or a phrase can help form a relationship with a patient in just a few minutes. By contrast, the wrong words or confusing body language can create a barrier between the patient and the physician.

In this section, I will discuss techniques derived from nearly 100 interviews with patients and families that will help you form a relationship in just a short period of time. Many of these practices were developed based on interviews with people who have experienced hearing bad news first-hand. These individuals readily shared what they felt and how they interpreted the words and body language of the physician.

A trusting relationship with a healthcare provider is the number one predictor of patient satisfaction and patient loyalty. (We will cover this more in depth when discussing enhancing the overall patient experience later in this book.) But with the increased demands on doctors and nurses to see more patients in shorter times, to document more, and simply go faster, many of my colleagues doubt whether it is possible in today's environment to build a relationship with a patient in less than five minutes. In fact, it has been shown that when done correctly, a healthcare provider can build trust in less than 60 seconds.[16] Primary care physicians who often have the opportunity to get to know a patient over a long period of time build relationships easier. But by using the techniques that follow, even medical providers meeting a patient for the first time can form a trusting relationship very quickly.

Relationship Words
Just a cog in the wheel

For almost 20 years, I routinely introduced myself to patients and families as "one of" the residents or doctors. After all, this is what I was taught, and it made sense because it was true. Medicine is a team sport, and we are supposed to promote the teamwork concept to the patient. For years, I mistakenly believed that by promoting the team approach, it gave patients comfort, knowing that their child had a large hospital with all its staff looking out for them. After years of research and interviewing patients and families, I learned I've been wrong. Time and time again, patients told me that their interpretation of this phrase was entirely different from what I expected. Introducing myself as "one of" the doctors caring for their baby immediately built an emotional obstacle between me and the family. From the patient's point of view, since I was only "one of" the doctors, there was little chance of building a one-on-one relationship.

The reality is that patients and families do not find comfort in a big institution. They seek a relationship with someone they can identify as their caregiver who will take responsibility for their treatment. A physician introducing himself as "one of the doctors" sends a signal that he/she is avoiding responsibility. It sends the message that he/she is just a small cog in a large wheel, so if anything goes wrong, they are not to blame. On the other hand, patients report feeling great comfort knowing that there is one physician who is taking responsibility for their care at that moment. The physician who introduces himself as "the one responsible" for a patient's care can immediately begin the trusting relationship that patients and families are seeking. Although it may be a surprise to healthcare workers, patients and families frequently express more confidence in their care when an intern introduces herself as "the intern who is responsible for their care" compared to a senior physician who introduces herself as "one of the doctors." Patients know that an intern is young and inexperienced, but they still find comfort in knowing the name of the person who will be their primary contact for that shift.

Pronouns – I can't have a relationship with a "We"

Pronouns have the power to start a one-on-one relationship or create a barrier by making a conversation less personal. Telling a patient that "We recommend treating your cancer in this manner" has a similar effect to "I am one of the doctors treating you." It diffuses any personal responsibility. "We" is a hard concept for a patient to grasp. Who is "We?" The hospital, your practice, or the insurance company? Changing the pronoun from "We" to "I" immediately establishes ownership, trust, and human connection. Simply stating, "What I recommend in this situation is…" immediately creates that one-on-one relationship with your patients.

The concept of "I" vs. "We" is especially important when discussing a serious or life-threatening diagnosis. After hearing that their world has just changed dramatically for the worse, the patient and family immediately need to know that there is an expert they can bond with and feel confident will help them through the next steps. As human beings, we cannot bond to "We." We can only bond to another individual.

I think, therefore, I don't know

Who among us wants a physician, nurse, or practitioner who is not sure of himself? Telling a patient and family that, after reviewing all of the lab tests, you think or you believe that they have a serious illness sounds perfectly legitimate. After all, we know that medicine is not an exact science, and there are almost always further tests that need to be done before a definite diagnosis can be made. Images in our minds of attorneys calling over a diagnosis that is not 100% accurate cause us to "hedge" our diagnosis out of self-preservation.

Hedging is even more common when giving bad news or having a difficult conversation. As human beings, we never want to upset someone, and since we may not be completely sure of a diagnosis, it makes sense to say "I think" or "maybe." The problem with these terms is that they suggest uncertainty, and patients and families need a doctor who is the absolute expert in the room. Uncertainty can result in strengthening the denial phase of grieving, or making patients and families angry that the doctor would say something that is so life changing without being totally sure. While we as doctors recognize that we do not know anything 100%, it is not the uncertainty that causes the problem. It is the word choice. Simply changing the words "I think" or "I believe" to "I am concerned" or "I am worried" conveys a very different message. Both phrases are uncertain. However, the doctor who "thinks" does not "know." In contrast, the doctor who "is concerned there is a brain tumor" is caring and compassionate. The latter conveys a very different message and strengthens the relationship. Patients want a doctor who is concerned about them.

As an example, let us look at two different ways of breaking the same news.

"Mr. Smith, I looked at your X-ray. There's a spot on your lung that I think may be cancer. I'd like to send you to an oncologist."

"Mr. Smith, 1 looked at your X-ray. There's a spot on your lung and I'm very concerned that it may be cancer. I'd like to send you to an oncologist."

Simply by changing one word, you went from a physician who does not know to a physician who is compassionate and invested in the patient. Not only are we doctors or nurses but we are real people who are genuinely caring and concerned for their well-being. We are worried about the outcome and their future health. So, those simple but powerful words, "worried" and "concerned," display your compassion and continue to strengthen the bond with the patient and family.

Don't speak in scripts—It's shallow

And finally, another phrase that can get in the way of forming a relationship or help to build one is the generic, "I'm here if you need anything." This is a script, and an empty sentence that is interpreted as, "I hope you don't call me." Instead, simply say, "I will help you get through this."

Avoiding difficult conversations about death is common not only from neighbors and friends, but for those of us who frequently encounter highly emotional situations on a regular basis. Throughout my career, I have seen physicians avoid the dying patient's room when the family is present. I have seen nurses make small talk while a loved one is dying. I have seen doctors avoid having end of life or hospice discussions until the disease has progressed far too long. Insurance allows patients to receive hospice care starting up to six months before they die, yet most physicians do not present it as an option to patients until much later. Why? Most physicians would say that they do not have the time or they do not want to make the patient sad. The truth is that it is human nature to avoid situations that are uncomfortable. As such, we either postpone the difficult conversation or avoid the topic altogether.

Often, we use social workers and chaplains during difficult times. They provide an essential and comforting service and help to put patients and families at ease. But it is important that when you bring in the social worker or the chaplain, you do not leave the room. Stay with them. You have already formed a relationship with them by saying that you are concerned or worried, so your presence further solidifies that bond.

Forming a relationship quickly

1.   Take personal responsibility. "I am the doctor responsible for your care today."

2.   Form a one-on-one relationship. Use "I," not "we."

3.   Don't speak in scripts. Be Genuine.

4.   Be there when it counts.

5.   Be silent when appropriate.

A—ACCOUNTABILITY

The Power of "personally"

After building a relationship, let the patient and family know that you are knowledgeable and in control. (Remember goals two and three of Breaking Bad News.) Use the statements we previously discussed, such as, "I know this is incredibly difficult news, but I will be with you and I will help you get through this." This is an extremely important point. As the one who delivered the crushing news, you have just changed their lives forever. You are now bonded with them and are in their minds for eternity.

Patients and families who have heard tragic news can remember every detail about it, so be accountable. Let the patient and family know you are not going anywhere and you will stay involved with their care. "I'm here and I know what to do." This is the time to let the patient and family know that they can figuratively drape their arms around your shoulders and you will lead them to the next step. This can be accomplished whether or not you are a primary care provider or an emergency medicine physician meeting a patient for the first time. Take just a few minutes to tell the patient that he/she will be transferred to the intensive care nursery but that you will "personally" make sure that everyone on the new team will know every detail about their case. This personal attention goes a long way in building that ever-important relationship.

Primary care physicians often assume that their patients will know that, although they were referred to a specialist, the primary doctor will still be involved with their care. This is not always the case. If you already have a long-standing relationship with a patient being referred to a specialist, assure the patient and family that you will stay involved and will be available to coordinate care.

Finally, any "special treatment" goes a long way. There is an old mantra that I repeatedly heard from my professors in medical school: it states, "Mother, Father, Sister, Brother." It means that physicians should treat all their patients as if they were their own family member. We all want to feel special, and patients are no different. Comfort your patient by a statement such as, "I know Dr. Smith very well and he has a great reputation. I would trust him with my health. When I am finished answering your questions, I will personally give him a call." By taking this initiative, you are being accountable to your patients and strengthening the relationship.

M—MEET AGAIN

Think about the last time you called customer service or tech support. After discussing your problem and reaching a solution, the representative will often end the discussion by asking if there is anything else they can help you with before hanging up. We all know that this is a scripted response that they are required to say to everyone. It's not sincere and gives us the impression that the representative is hoping that we say no so they can move on to the next customer. Scripted and vague statements are always perceived as insincere. Patients have a similar impression when a doctor or nurse tells them to call if they need anything. It's a script. When we say "have a nice day" or "hope you feel better" to someone, it's similar to what the customer service agent says on the phone. During difficult times, people find comfort in clarity and sincerity. Be specific about the next steps and when you will be back by saying, "I will be back to check on you in a few hours" or "You're going to see the specialist but I want you to make an appointment to see me in two weeks. In the meantime, I want you to promise to call if you have any questions or problems." Being specific and avoiding scripts will solidify that relationship and make your patient feel as if they will not be abandoned. By telling them exactly when you will meet again, you're giving them the comfort they really need at that moment.

Using the BBN P.R.O.G.R.A.M principles covered in this section will not only provide sufficient guidance for anyone giving bad news, but will also aid in helping patients and families when they need it the most. It can make the difference between uncertainty and acceptance. Patients and families will remember the healthcare provider with appreciation and fondness even during the most tragic time of their lives.

This is a good time to review the three goals of Breaking Bad News:

1. The patient and family should feel that their physician understands their situation and is genuinely compassionate.

2. The patient and family should feel that their physician is the expert in the room and trust that they will lead them to the next step.

3. The patient and family should feel that their

physician will not abandon them.

Following Up and Debriefing

As a neonatologist, when the sad death of a baby occurs in the NICU, it is extremely important that the parents do not feel that they are being abandoned. The same is true for any death, young or old. The unimaginable has just occurred, and the family must know specifically what will happen next. I frequently ask parents after their baby has died if it is okay for me to call them in a few days. I also tell them that they will likely have questions in the near future. Then I give them my card and encourage them to make an appointment to talk later when they are ready. It is my experience that most parents accept the invitation.

During the follow-up visit, I answer as many of the family's questions as possible. Many physicians avoid this type of conversation, fearing that they will likely not have answers to many of the questions that will be asked. Medicine is not an exact science and we frequently don't know all the answers. However, it's perfectly acceptable to respond by saying, "I don't have the answer for you right now and often we don't know, but I can promise you that I will do whatever I can to help you find the answers you are seeking. If I do get an answer, you will be the first person I call."

This follow-up conversation and debriefing solidifies the relationship that hopefully has already been formed with the family. They should leave feeling that the physician and hospital are not hiding anything and are confident that everything possible was done to help the patient and the family. The healthcare professionals who have guided them through the worst time of their lives have formed an indelible mark in the minds of the family.

The Donut Effect

I heard a lecture from a social worker many years ago and he referred to what he called "The Donut Effect." I had seen it many times but never thought much about it until I heard someone give it a name. Sadly, newborn babies often die without ever leaving the hospital. The only home they knew was an incubator or crib in a NICU. Some babies die after a few days. Others die after months of battling complication after complication. In both instances, the NICU is the place that the parents visited every day. Even after a death, it is the place they feel closest to their baby.

By anyone's standards, the NICU is a special place. Doctors and nurses care for the smallest patients while simultaneously helping the parents through the most stressful and scariest time of their lives. When a baby is critically ill, there is a special bond that occurs between the parents and the nurses, doctors, and staff who care for the baby. I thank God every day for the opportunity to work with such an amazing group of people. But with all of the magical moments that occur, there is also a lot of sadness. Tragically, babies die, despite the best care of these fragile patients. When that happens, it affects everyone, but for most of us who have not experienced it first-hand, the pain the parents feel is unimaginable.

It is not unusual for parents to visit the NICU weeks or even months after the death of their baby with the stated intention of thanking the doctors, nurses, and staff for all the care and compassion they received while their baby was ill. When visiting, they often bring a token expression of their appreciation such as donuts. It is a time for closure, a time for hugs, and a time for a few tears. Only the astute observer, however, will notice the frequent and subtle glances by the parents toward the room where their baby died. This is what has been so appropriately called, The Donut Effect. Parents use the donuts and the excuse of thanking the staff as a reason to visit the place they feel most connected with their baby. Much in the same way people visit cemeteries to feel close to their deceased loved ones, parents feel closest to their baby when they are in "their room" in the NICU. This can also occur with adults or older children who have prolonged hospital stays.

So the next time a family visits the hospital to thank the staff or bring a gift after a loved one has passed, watch to see whether they are looking in the direction of the room. If they are, ask them if they would like to go in for a visit. It's been my experience that the answer is frequently, yes. Sitting in the room quietly, as if by a gravestone, is often therapeutic.

Key Points

1.   Be specific on when you will see them again.

2.   Follow up with a phone call after
       delivering tragic news.

3.   Encourage patients and families to
       return with questions.

Chapter 4

Communication and Enhancing the Patient Experience

My grandmother died when she was 93 years old. Until her death, she never would agree to go to a hospital. She used to say that everyone she knew who had died, did so in a hospital. Therefore, it was logical to her that if she never went to a hospital she would live forever. It turns out that my grandmother was correct: the first time she was ever admitted to a hospital she died. Of course, it was merely a coincidence, but most people die in hospitals. In her own simple way, what my grandmother was really saying was that hospitals are scary places that make us feel vulnerable and out of control. They require us to put our care in the hands of people whom we've just met. The reality is that regardless of how excellent the care is or how pleasant the stay, even if everything goes perfectly, no one actually enjoys being in a hospital. When was the last time you heard someone say that they loved the time they spent in the hospital? As medical professionals, our goal is simple: to provide excellent healthcare while doing whatever we can to make a patient's stay as comfortable as possible. Considering that patients are in a strange place, subjected to a battery of tests and needles, and anxious about the disease that put them in the hospital in the first place, this is no easy task. But by utilizing proper communication skills that put patients at ease and by following five key principles addressed in Chapter 5, we can help patients have the best experience as possible.

Until this point, we have discussed the BBN P.R.O.G.R.A.M with respect to the communication skills necessary to break bad news to patients and families. These same communication techniques are also effective for building rapport with a patient, navigating through a difficult conversation, or improving the experience of a patient in the hospital. Communication is the basis of all relationships and is the number one predictor of patient satisfaction. The healthcare professional who learns how to communicate well will not only be able to navigate difficult dialogues with confidence but will also possess the skills required to build a successful practice and to help all of their patients during sickness and wellness. Good communicators also make better leaders, work more synergistically with staff, and are better equipped to build strong relationships in both their professional and private life. Let's explore how communicating well can significantly help patients when they need us the most.

The Truth About Patient Satisfaction Scores

"Understanding is the first step to acceptance and only with acceptance can there be recovery." – J.K. Rowling

Currently, patient satisfaction is easily the hottest topic in medicine. It affects reimbursement, hospital census, and is absolutely essential for any healthcare system to compete in today's market. While this book is not intended to be a comprehensive review of patient satisfaction surveys, it is necessary that every medical provider has a basic understanding of the topic and dispel some common myths. In a survey by

The Beryl Institute, an organization dedicated to improving the patient experience, 90% of consumers stated that patient experience was extremely/very important to them and will significantly affect their future healthcare decisions.[17] Press Ganey, one of the largest administrators of patient satisfaction surveys, found that providing a good patient experience is five times more likely to influence brand loyalty than other marketing strategies.[18] Although patient experience is critical to the success of any healthcare system, most doctors and nurses don't fully understand what patient satisfaction scores are, how they are measured, and why they are so important. Following are the basics of patient satisfaction surveys and some common myths and misconceptions.

Patient Satisfaction 101

For decades, hospitals have utilized patient surveys as a measure of consumer satisfaction primarily for internal tracking and marketing purposes. The federal government first became active in patient satisfaction in 2001, and by 2006, the Hospital Consumer Assessment of Healthcare Providers and Systems (HCAHPS) (pronounced "H-caps") became the first standardized national patient survey on hospital care. The survey, developed by the Centers for Medicaid and Medicare Services (CMS) is sent to inpatients after discharge to obtain feedback about their level of satisfaction with the care they received. In 2005, hospitals began receiving financial incentives for participating in surveys. These financial incentives were further strengthened in 2012, when CMS established criteria that would reward or penalize hospitals and doctors by their performance.[19] With the growing popularity of websites that allow patients to rate their doctors and hospitals, providing a good patient experience has become exceedingly important. Simply put, patient satisfaction affects all aspects of healthcare, especially the bottom line.

According to a report by Deloitte in May 2018, hospitals with excellent HCAHPS scores had a net margin of 4.7% on average, as compared to a net margin of just 1.8% for hospitals with low ratings. The report also found that comparing hospitals in the same market region and adjusting for hospital characteristics, a 10% point increase in the number of respondents giving the hospital a 9 or 10 (a "top box") is associated with a higher net margin of 1.4%.[20] In addition, Press Ganey found that hospitals receiving the top 25% of patient satisfaction scores tended to also fall within the top 25% in profitability. Of interest is that the higher profitability is only partly due to differences in reimbursement. In fact, reimbursement makes up only 25% of the difference. The remaining 75% comes from patient loyalty and a robust referral base that occurs when patients are satisfied with their care. The obvious conclusion is that today's patient generally chooses their hospital or doctor through recommendations rather than quality of care.[18]

The financial ramifications of patient satisfaction scores, especially in today's ultra-competitive healthcare system are extremely important to hospital administrators. However, to physicians and nurses directly caring for patients, there are more important reasons to improve patient satisfaction than financial incentives. Despite the economic pressures, most healthcare providers are in the business of healing and are more motivated by their altruistic views than financial incentives, especially when those incentives are more heavily weighted toward hospitals and not personal reimbursement. After all is said and done, I believe that the majority of medical professionals who dedicate their lives to healing the sick would agree that improving a patient's experience is, at its core, simply the right thing to do.

What most don't realize is that patient satisfaction is also strongly associated with better treatment compliance, improved outcomes, and reduced length of stay.[10, 21-23] Furthermore, high patient satisfaction is related to increased loyalty, a significant reduction in malpractice lawsuits, and even reduced professional burnout.[24] In summary, enhancing the patient experience has far-reaching benefits. It's no wonder that more than 80% of hospital executives list improving the patient experience in the top three of their most important objectives.[25]

Improved Patient Satisfaction

- Improved patient compliance with treatment plan

- Better patient outcomes

- Reduction of malpractice claims

- Reduction in professional burnout

Myths and Misperceptions

There are many misconceptions about HCAHPS and patient satisfaction surveys. Most of the misinformation has fallen into the convenient narrative that patient reviews are beyond the control of the provider. It is true that it is not a perfect system. Some studies even suggest that physicians may feel pressure to practice less than optimal medicine for fear they will be rated poorly on their survey.[26] All things considered, the overwhelming consensus is that a good patient experience leads to improved compliance, better outcomes, and reduced malpractice claims.

Before committing to providing the best possible experience for our patients, it is essential that everyone involved in patient care understands the basics of how surveys are performed. This book is not intended to be a comprehensive authority on HCAHPS and satisfaction surveys. However, I believe that it is important to dispel a few common misconceptions about the topic that are often used as excuses for lower scores.

Myth #1: Patient satisfaction has little to do with clinical outcomes.

In 2008, Jha et al. published a study in the New England Journal of Medicine in which the researchers concluded that a patient's positive experience in a hospital is linked to excellent clinical care, reduced medical errors, and advanced performance outcomes.[21] Since then, there have been multiple studies showing a positive correlation between satisfaction surveys and clinical outcomes. In 2013, Doyle et al. reviewed 55 studies and found that the large majority showed a positive relationship between patient experience and self-rated and objectively measured health outcomes.[10] And, according to the 2018 Deloitte study mentioned earlier, the hospitals with the top 25% of HCAHPS scores are also in the top 25% in clinical outcomes. Press Ganey found similar results.[27] To be fair, there have been published studies that have shown little or no relationship between HCAHPS results and the quality of care delivered.[28-30] The far majority, however, support the theory that when patients have a better experience and trust their healthcare provider, they are more likely to follow the treatment plan, are more compliant with their medications, and are more likely to follow up with their physician.

Myth #2: Very few patients fill out satisfaction surveys.

The average HCAHPS response rate has decreased from 33% in 2008 to 28% in 2016.[31]

At first glance, that may seem low, but when we put it into perspective, the response rate in healthcare is generally on par or slightly higher than the average response rate of almost every other industry. More people fill out their satisfaction surveys for hospitals than for hotels, airlines, or car dealerships. I believe this is most likely due to the relative importance we place on healthcare compared to non-healthcare products or services.

Myth #3: Only unhappy patients fill out their survey.

On average, 60-70% of responding patients rated their hospitals in the top box, a 9 or 10 on a scale of 0–10. Additionally, 70% of patients nationally said they would definitely recommend their hospital to friends and family and the average star rating for doctors was 4 out of 5 stars.[32]

It is also a common misperception that happy people don't take the time to make comments on surveys. According to Press Ganey, approximately one-third to one-half of responding patients took the time to add comments to their inpatient surveys. When we more closely analyze who commented, we see that 47% of patients who gave medium ratings made a comment, 59% who gave low ratings took the time to place a comment, and 45% of people who gave high ratings commented on their surveys. So for the most part, those who make comments are evenly distributed between those who gave low, medium, and high ratings.[27]

Myth #4: I just don't have the time.

I often hear from healthcare professionals that with all the added demands placed on them, such as electronic medical records and the increased pressure to see more and more patients, they just don't have the time for lengthy discussions with their patients or their families anymore. I am frequently told that this all sounds very nice, but given the time restraints on doctors, making that kind of personal connection is simply not possible. Emergency medicine physicians especially bring up this concern. But the fact is, the manner in which we communicate is even more important during very short encounters with patients and families whom we have not met before. And believe it or not, using the correct words and providing a consistent message in the right manner is actually more time-efficient. If you do it incorrectly, it will result in more questions, more anger, and take a lot more time.

A key mistake hospitals, corporations, and offices make is putting efficiency in front of courtesy. When efficiency is the top priority, courtesy and compassion will always suffer. When compassion is placed first, efficiency will almost always follow. It turns out your mother was right; doing it right the first time will eventually save time.

Hospitals Are Not Hotels— Charlie Brown and the Football

For years, the healthcare industry has recognized that many doctors and nurses lack the necessary communication skills to convey their natural compassion and form relationships with patients and families. Analyses of HCAHPS scores frequently show that physicians receive poor grades for their ability to communicate. Of course, there are exceptions to the rule. I know many physicians who have excellent bedside manner and a great ability to communicate, but the bottom line is, when you analyze patient satisfaction scores, physicians and nurses often receive poor grades on their communication skills.

Trying to address this problem, hospitals and other types of healthcare systems turned to the hotel industry as a model. Since the 1980s, and at the advice of third party consultants, hospital employees were asked to behave as if patients were customers in a resort. They were handed pre-packaged programs taken from the training books of hotels and were provided personal coaches, frequently with no medical experience, to tell them how to interact with a patient. Nurses, staff, and physicians were fed pre-formatted scripts. They were instructed on what to say when greeting a patient and again when leaving the room, often asking them to repeat the same hospital motto with each and every encounter. Risk management departments gave classes on how to resolve conflict and provided a list of specific "Dos" and "Don'ts" when having discussions with an unhappy patient. Unfortunately, this resulted in little or no improvement in patient satisfaction. Their plan failed miserably.

Shocked at the results, many hospitals doubled down on their theory and continued to mimic the hotel and vacation industry even more. Walls were painted brighter colors. Spas were installed in labor and delivery units, WiFi and televisions were placed everywhere. To both the hospitals and the hotel executives giving the advice, the theory seemed sound: make the hospital nice and beautiful and patients will have a better experience. Once again, the results were disappointing. No matter how many times this approach has failed in the past, hospitals continue to make the same mistakes over and over again: treating hospitals as if they were hotels. As Einstein once said, "The definition of insanity is doing the same thing over and over again and expecting different results." I often feel as if I am watching Charlie Brown trying to kick the football, thinking that if he just tried one more time, Lucy won't pull the ball away.

Many hospitals continue to fail to see the bigger picture. They forget that there is a major difference between a hospital and a hotel. Guests stay in a hotel because they choose to be there. Patients stay in a hospital because they must be there. Hotel guests seek comfort and the amenities of home. Patients, on the other hand, seek the care and kindness of other people. They hunger for human interaction in a time of vulnerability. It's a trusting relationship that is sought by patients, not a comfortable chair or Netflix on demand. Patients in hospitals are nervous and unhappy about their circumstances. Most have little or no knowledge of medicine and they are forced to put their lives in the hands of doctors, nurses, and staff. Remember, no one chooses to be in a hospital. Healthcare is much more personal than a hotel, and the stakes are much higher. Patients do not want to be spoken to in scripts or repeated mottos. They don't want to receive information about their disease written on tri-fold handouts like brochures for local excursions. This approach is perceived as shallow and insincere. What patients really want is to connect with the people who are caring for them on a human-to-human basis. They want a relationship with their healthcare provider based on mutual respect. Scripts, handouts, and long wait times place barriers to meaningful relationships. There is nothing wrong with hospitals adding benefits such as satellite TV, WiFi, and spas, but these types of amenities are consistently poor predictors of the overall patient experience. Without trust and respect between patients and their healthcare providers, a bad experience is almost certain regardless of how pretty the walls are painted.

This is not to suggest that communication is the only factor determining the patient experience, but it is certainly the foundation. As hospitals found out the hard way, without meaningful communication with the goal of doctor and nurse-to-patient bonding, a good patient experience is unlikely. As with any building, fixing the roof and the windows before the foundation is futile. If hospitals do not provide the resources to train their staff how to communicate effectively and with compassion, the same mistakes of the past will be repeated.

Building Patient Loyalty

How do we define a "positive patient experience?" According to the Hospitals Care Research Network, "having a high-quality interaction with their healthcare provider who makes patients feel that they are respected and listened to, that their opinions are taken into consideration and valued, is more important to patients than having a lengthy visit with their provider."[33]

It is clear that the ability of a healthcare professional to form a relationship with their patients is the best predictor of a patient's overall experience. Let's examine what really counts. In two separate studies by Press-Ganey (2003 and

2011), surveyors looked at the top five predictors of patient loyalty.[27] In the chart below, I have taken the liberty to place an asterisk next to each of the top predictors that are directly or indirectly related to communication. Notice that every single predictor has an asterisk. According to the two surveys, patient loyalty is totally dependent on communication skills.

Top Predictors of Patient Loyalty

2003	2011
How well staff worked together to care for you*	Response to your concerns during your hospital stay*
Overall cheerfulness of the hospital*	Degree which staff addressed your emotional needs*
How well staff responded to your concerns*	Staff's effort to include you in decisions*
Amount of attention paid to your personal needs*	How well the nurses kept you informed*
Staff insensitivity to inconvenience of hospitalization*	Promptness to responding to call button*

Notice what is missing from this table. There is no mention of outcomes. There is no mention of wait times in the emergency department, the quality of the food, or aesthetics of the rooms. More recent studies have shown that little has changed. In 2018, Press Ganey reported that the top three predictors of "most likely to recommend" were again all related to communication and respect. Yet, hospitals continue to make the same mistakes over and over again, putting the majority of their resources into making their system more efficient and easier to navigate. They pay companies handsomely to print out information sheets explaining just about every disease and medicine to the patients, believing that an informed patient is a happy and loyal patient. It is really quite simple. If you connect to a patient by treating them with respect and making them feel as if they are genuinely cared for, they will have a good experience.

If hospitals took the time to listen to patients and ask them what is important to them, they would start to understand what patients really need. They would come to the same conclusion every time: it's all in the delivery.

The Beryl Institute defines patient experience as "the sum of all interactions, shaped by an organization's culture, that influence patient perceptions across the continuum of care." It starts from the moment someone arrives at the hospital or doctor's office and lasts until they have settled back into their homes after discharge. Everything counts, from beginning to end. It is all about perception. Did the patient feel as if they were in a place where skilled people cared for them? Did they feel as if they were respected or did they feel like an inconvenience? The goal of every doctor, every nurse, and every hospital should always be to make patients feel like a welcomed guest, not like a visitor. Yet, hospitals unknowingly send patients subtle messages that they are indeed outsiders. They post rules and regulations and position signs throughout the building telling people where to sit and how to act. Patients and family members are handed "welcome" packets, which are immediately perceived by a frightened and unhappy patient as nothing more than a list of hospital policies that must be followed.

Of course, hospitals need rules and guidelines to protect the patients and their staff, but it's how they are delivered that counts. The "It's All in the Delivery" concept is not just about how we speak and communicate. It applies to every sign, every handout, and every encounter. To someone reading this book from the comfort of their own home, the concept of a poorly worded sign or a few rules causing patients to feel unwelcome may, at first, seem trivial. But as my grandmother pointed out in her own way, hospitals are scary places, and when people are frightened, their sensitivities are heightened. Things that normally would not be noticed are suddenly disconcerting and irritating.

For example, putting a sign above the sink at the entrance of a NICU asking parents to "Wash Your Hands Before Entering the Room" is a reasonable request. Babies are more susceptible to infection, and handwashing significantly reduces infections in sick babies. To a frightened parent visiting the nursery, however, this sign feels more like an order or just another hospital rule that must be followed before being allowed to see their own baby. Perhaps, it even suggests that the parents are too stupid to know that washing their hands before visiting is a good thing. Through my decades of interviewing patients and families, I have often been surprised about how even the most apparent innocuous signs can be misinterpreted by an emotional patient. Considering the "It's All in the Delivery" concept, let's think about how the hand washing sign could be rephrased. I came across this sign in a NICU one day. With a picture of a cute baby, it stated:

"It's true that I possess irresistible charm.
I understand how cute I am and you can't wait to see me.
But please don't forget to wash your hands. Germs can do me harm."

The next time you pass a sign in the hallway of your office or hospital, think about how the message might be interpreted by a patient or family. Imagining how the sign will be interpreted by a frightened patient or family member is the first step. Later in this chapter, we will review some of the hospital signs that I have seen and how they can send different and often conflicting messages to patients and families.

This Is Not Your Mother's Hospital Anymore

Until recently, it was common for friends and family to recommend a doctor with a poor bedside manner provided he/she were clinically capable. This is no longer the case for today's patient who expects more than just clinical competency. The modern patient demands a relationship with their healthcare provider based on mutual respect. Patients view themselves as consumers in control of their own health and free to spend their healthcare dollars wherever they feel is best. No longer is poor communication tolerated at the expense of good medical care. There is certainly no lack of resources for patients to make informed decisions. The internet provides easy access to a host of third party companies who rate hospitals by their clinical outcomes. Hospitals pay large sums of money to become certified and market themselves as excellent in various categories. However, the information is difficult to interpret and often overwhelming. One hospital is designated as Magnet Certified® another ranked higher by *U.S. News and Health Report*®. Others are Baby Friendly® or LeapFrog® certified. In the end, these rankings play a small role in a patient's choice. Even with all of the available data third parties provide, patients are still more likely to choose a hospital or healthcare provider through recommendations of friends or family.

A past statement by the executive staff at Kaiser Permanente, one of the nation's largest managed care consortia, declared, "Patients are less concerned with how much their physicians know than how much they care." The *Wall Street Journal* stated in a more recent article that "today's patient places more importance on doctors' interpersonal skills than their medical experience."

With limited funds available and the economic strains felt throughout the healthcare industry, hospitals would be better served investing in the patient experience instead of marketing or accumulating certifications that mean little to the average person. In fact, it has been estimated that one dollar spent improving patient satisfaction is equivalent to five dollars spent on marketing.[18] The smart executive should place more dollars into enhancing the patient experience.

Positive experiences come from extraordinary personal encounters. One bad encounter can negate all the positives. Building an exceptional patient experience is like playing baseball. It's a team sport, but each player comes to bat one at a time. For instance, when a patient comes to the emergency room, he or she is greeted by the receptionist who has an opportunity to create a positive encounter with a new patient. If that goes well, the triage nurse is next at bat and must communicate well to build on the connection the receptionist made. Next up might be the nurse and then doctor, each with a chance to add to the patient's overall experience—each having the opportunity to use their communication skills to form a relationship with the patient and their family. If any team member along the way does not communicate well and fails to contribute, the work of all of the rest is negated. Therefore, it's absolutely essential to achieve an exceptional experience that everyone communicates well, no matter what the situation may be.

Compassion Over Efficiency

Hospitals assume that by making the process of seeing a doctor less time consuming, patients will be happier. They forget that patients are not the same as customers. An auto repair shop has customers. Going to the auto shop and getting your oil changed would certainly be more satisfying if the process was faster. But patients want more than just efficiency. Patients want compassion. Although efficiency is important, compassion is almost always the victim of efficiency.

Yet hospitals continue to emphasize speed over clinical excellence or patient loyalty. Their solutions are almost always centered around technology such as placing laptops in examination rooms or asking physicians to carry tablets, encouraging them to multitask. In fact, multitasking actually slows down progress and risks medical errors.

Multitasking is actually a myth. It is well accepted that the human brain cannot perform two simultaneous tasks at one time unless one or more of the tasks are done automatically, such as walking and chewing gum. Attempting to multitask is actually switching our thoughts back and forth between two or more tasks, thereby increasing the chance of error.[34-36]

While some mistakenly believe that multitasking is necessary to get things done in a timely manner, from a patient's point of view, doctors and nurses who multitask are perceived as not paying attention to their needs. The popularity of electronic medical records has added to the problem, encouraging the medical professional to sit in front of a computer or tablet while listening to a patient with the promise of increased efficiency and better access to data. This has further driven a wedge into the human to human interaction that patients crave. Doctors and nurses attempting to type and listen at the same time will likely miss the nuances of what was said, especially those found in the subtleties of body language. Patients are likely to believe that the physician is preoccupied and doesn't feel compassion. This will lead to distrust, frustration, and a disconnect between the patient and physician.

In the end, multitasking will result in a longer interaction and increased number of mistakes. Patients will feel the doctor or nurse is not listening and are likely to ask more questions or repeat themselves, resulting in even a longer interaction. Patients may even become angry. Neither efficiency nor compassion is achieved.

Communication Rule #7: Place compassion over efficiency. It will save time.

On the other hand, when healthcare providers place courtesy and compassion first, efficiency will almost always follow. Sitting down and listening to the patient, as Dr. Falchuk did with Anne Dodge, will likely result in less questions, more effective communication, and actually save time. Over decades of teaching communication to healthcare providers, I have found this to be the most difficult concept for physicians and nurses to accept. Attempts at convincing healthcare professionals that sitting down and listening while avoiding multitasking actually takes less time, are often met with skepticism. I can promise you, however, that it is 100% true. Two years ago, my team trained the staff in one of the world's largest Neonatal Intensive Care Units with an average of 1,700 admissions each year and a capacity of 142 beds. The hospital delivers more than 15,000 babies each year. The NICU is busy, to say the least. The entire team of doctors, nurses, receptionists, and therapists were trained using the "It's All in the Delivery" communication techniques. The training program resulted in a 60%

increase in overall patient satisfaction ranking and more than 100% increase in physician communication scores. More importantly, there was no evidence that efficiency suffered at all. In fact, many of the physicians and practitioners reported increased efficiency due to less complaints.

Sitting Saves Time

A study by K.J. Swayden examined perceived time by patients when physicians and nurses sat down compared to standing up.[37] In this study, the average actual time each doctor sat in a patient's room was almost identical (1 minute, 4 seconds sitting vs. 1 minute 24 seconds standing). Patients were then asked to guess how much time the doctors spent in the room. Although the actual time spent in the room was the same, patients perceived that the doctors who sat down were in the room significantly longer (5 minutes, 14 seconds vs. 3 minutes, 40 seconds).

The next time you enter a patient's room, mark the time on your watch. Sit down and speak with your patient and family using the communication techniques reviewed in the next section. Then do your physical exam. Record the time you were in the room. For your next visit, enter the room and attempt to multitask and then compare the time spent. I believe you'll find out for yourself that spending quality time by focusing on the patient will make you more efficient, save time, and increase patient satisfaction.

Key Learning Points

- Positive experiences come from extraordinary encounters.

- One bad encounter can negate many positives.

- Patient experience starts and ends with communication—single best predictor.

Chapter 5

The Five Principles of Communication for a Positive Patient Experience

During my lifelong quest to become a better communicator, I have identified five basic principles of communication that contribute to a positive patient experience. As a physician, I have learned that keeping these techniques in mind, as we interact with those in our care, will result in the best possible experience for our patients and their families. Whether the interaction is routine or tragic, these principles will help promote relationship-building and convey compassion. To be clear, these are what I believe are general communication principles that apply equally to professional and personal life. No matter what the circumstances, understanding the five basic principles of communication will help anyone navigate through even the most difficult dialogues.

Principle #1: It's all in the delivery.

It comes down to this most fundamental of tenets—how you say something is more important than what you say. Every word has both a definition and a connotation that evokes a unique feeling to the person receiving it. This is further amplified when emotions are running high. Patients are rarely happy about going to the doctor and even more unhappy about being admitted to the hospital. They are not at their best. Words, that under normal circumstances would be considered innocuous, might suddenly cause an adverse response. It is the skilled communicator who considers every word and how it is delivered before speaking.

Before starting an interaction with someone, think about what you want to say and how you want to say it. Use the proper body language for the message you would like to convey. For example, does this situation call for a lighter mood or is the news tragic? Is the patient over-anxious about a minor illness? If so, perhaps a smile and reassuring tone is appropriate. Or, will the message be serious and require a different approach? These things must be considered in each circumstance. As a colleague of mine often says, "Before entering the room, stop and take your own pulse." Take a few moments to calm down and think about how you want to deliver the message. The conversations will go much more smoothly, help you form a trusting relationship with the patient, and still save you time.

In addition to verbal and non-verbal language, the tone, cadence, and inflection of the words spoken must also be considered in order to avoid seeming insensitive or rude. A rapid cadence, for instance, is often interpreted by the listener as rushed and anxious. On the other hand, the proper use of pauses at critical times transmit feelings of compassion and sensitivity toward the situation. Remember that serious discussions require more serious time commitments. While they may take a while, doing it right will save time in the long run.

Understanding the significance of how a message is delivered is half the battle. This basic knowledge of communication, combined with the use of imagination and a good plan, will significantly improve your ability to have effective dialogue with patients and form a trusting relationship almost instantly.

Forming a relationship with patients starts the moment they arrive at the hospital or office. Well before the physicians, nurses, and staff have had an opportunity to interact on a human to human basis, patients have already begun to form an opinion. Long wait times and inefficient systems only make patients more anxious, even before seeing a doctor or nurse. It is the responsibility of the hospital to set the tone for the visit from the beginning. Yet hospital administrators not well versed in how messages are delivered continue to be their own worst enemy. Fancy slogans about excellence in care and dedication to their patients are no substitute for making someone feel as if they are an invited guest. Hospitals like to advertise that they treat every patient as if they were a guest but then send subliminal and overt messages to patients that they are, instead, visitors who must abide by their rules.

Let's review some common examples of signs hospitals believe are necessary but can quickly send the wrong message.

Picture 1:

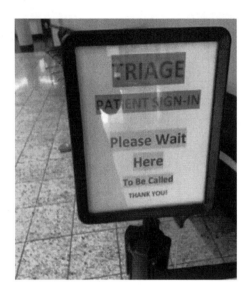

At first glance, this is a fairly innocent and straightforward sign, but how is it interpreted by an anxious patient who just arrived in the emergency department? What message does it give to the family members concerned about a loved one who was just brought to the hospital by ambulance? Putting aside for the moment that the sign looks like a ransom note from the Lindbergh kidnapping, it is short and cold and doesn't take into consideration the circumstances and the state of mind of the person reading it. As the saying goes: there is no second chance to make a first impression. The sign is clearly not an inviting "welcome" but rather an order interpreted as "sign your name, sit down, and wait to be called." Is this something you would put on the front door of your home? Of course not.

There are numerous ways to rephrase this sign to make a patient feel like a welcome guest. One example is the following:

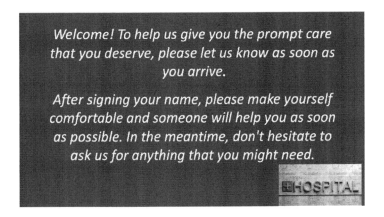

Picture 2:

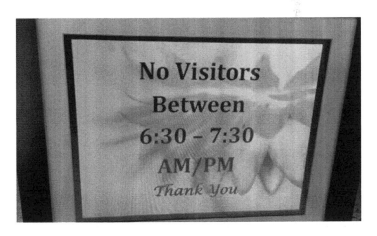

After being told where to wait, patients are commonly asked to fill out numerous forms only to be told again where to sit to wait some more. After getting past the first obstacle, the patient is subjected to more signs explaining various rules about refraining from eating or informing them when they cannot visit. The sign in Picture 2 was clearly written by someone who did not consider the delivery. It doesn't tell family members the hours they can visit, only when they cannot. The

natural question that most people have after reading the sign is, "Why can't we visit during those times?" To doctors, nurses, and staff, the answer is obvious: shift change. In order to protect the patients' privacy, families are asked to wait outside while the nurses discuss each patient. This is not at all apparent to those who are unfamiliar with the flow of hospitals. Therefore, the imagination of the nervous patient or family member immediately wonders what happens during the hours they may not visit, and their thoughts may become irrational. Careful consideration of how to treat patients and families as welcome guests would have been useful before posting this sign.

This is a better way to phrase the sign:

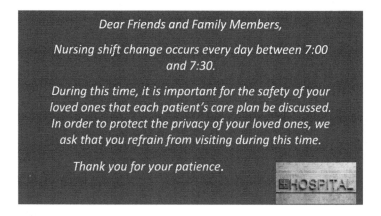

This sign would promote a message of partnership and clarity instead of distrust and being adversarial.

Picture 3 is particularly amusing to me.

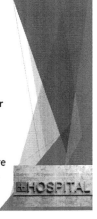

Patients and Families

We are committed to providing a safe environment
for the care of you and your family

This hospital has a

Zero Tolerance Policy for Abusive or Violent Behavior
toward
Our team members, patients, and visitors.

Thank you for helping us provide safe and effective care

Before placing this sign in the emergency department waiting room, hospital administrators should have asked themselves what percentage of patients will be abusive to their staff and if that small percentage is likely to be dissuaded from exhibiting abusive behavior simply by reading a sign. Does anyone believe that someone who is about to become violent or verbally abusive will read this sign and immediately become civil? Of course not. For the other 98% of patients who are unlikely to become abusive, the sign only results in a clear message that the hospital does not believe patients can be trusted to act in a respectful manner. It further establishes that patients and family members are just visitors who will be asked to leave if the rules are not followed. Of course, hospitals need to have rules for the safety of everyone, but being more aware of the underlying message that is being delivered will help to phrase signs that make patients feel more like guests. A good rule of thumb is to ask yourself: Is this a sign I would place in my home?

Questions to ask before placing a sign

1.   Does the sign make patients and families feel like guests?

2.   Does the sign promote a feeling of mutual trust and respect?

3.   Does the sign help patients and family members navigate the system?

4.   Does the sign explain the reason for the rule?

5.   Is the sign necessary or can it be replaced by human interaction?

In addition to poor presentation and word choices on signs, there are other seemingly harmless actions that deliver the wrong and impersonal message. The simple act of shutting a patient's door, for example, can be interpreted the wrong way if communication techniques are not considered. In Fred Lee's book, he gives the following example of how shutting a door can illicit many different emotions in patients. The following scenario is paraphrased from *If Disney Ran Your Hospital*, by Fred Lee, and the responses are modified using the "It's All in the Delivery" techniques.[8]

A frequent problem patients encounter, especially if their rooms are near the nurse's station, is that it often gets loud during shift change. Depending on the nurse's knowledge of communication principles, the problem can be handled in one of three possible ways.

Bad — The nurse does not shut the door. She is oblivious to the noise or just does not get up to close the door. The patient does not get their needed rest, which will likely result in an unhappy patient who believes the nurses are inconsiderate to his/her situation and do not care if they get sleep.

Better — Realizing that the hallway is getting noisy, the nurse shuts the patient's door. On the surface, this seems like a considerate thing to do. The vulnerable or anxious patient, however, may wonder why the door was shut and may allow their mind to wonder. Perhaps the nurses are discussing their case and information is being withheld. Or maybe the daytime nurse is telling the night nurse that the patient asked to go to the bathroom too many times and is needy. Shutting the door may have been a considerate gesture by the nurse, but without communication, it leaves the possibility that more questions will be raised later.

Best — Realizing that the hallway is getting noisy, the nurse who understands the principles of good communication shuts the door with an explanation. "Mr. Jones, we sometimes get a little noisy during shift change. We don't get to see each other very often and may not realize how loud we can get. So if it is okay with you, I am going to shut your door. I will open it when the shift change is over if you would like."

Let's analyze this version using the "It's All in the Delivery" communication principles. In this example, the nurse accomplishes several things in a brief, four-sentence inter-action. First, she explains to Mr. Jones why she is shutting the door, avoiding any possibility that he will misinterpret the action as deceitful. Second, the nurse has conveyed the message that she and her colleagues like each other. This promotes a sense of teamwork. Finally, by admitting they get loud, the nurse portrays her and the other nurses as real people who enjoy working and caring for their patients. This establishes the nurses as genuine people. This will be discussed further during principle number two.

Principle #2: It's hard to fire your best friends.

My mother always told me, "Anthony, it's hard to fire your best friend." No matter how successful I became, my mother would still push her best friend philosophy on me. I used to think, why is she so afraid that I would get fired? It wasn't until much later in my career when I became more aware of how physicians and patients communicate that I finally un-derstood what she meant. She wasn't talking about getting fired or becoming friends with my boss. She was telling me in her own way that it is always important to take the time to become everyone's best friend. Best friends trust each other. They confide in each other and have an open dialogue. Best friends forgive each other when something doesn't go right, and most of all, best friends stay loyal. Wouldn't it be great if patients could have that type of relationship with their doctors and nurses, even if meeting for the first time? My mother's advice also holds true for both the routine and the difficult conversations. Patients are more likely to listen to and follow the advice of physicians with whom they have a friendly relationship.

Although the "G" in the BBN P.R.O.G.R.A.M acronym as it relates to breaking bad news, stands for "Gradual," when the acronym refers to more routine patient interactions, the "G" stands for "Genuine." Being a genuine person is an essential ingredient for establishing rapport with someone and rapport is the basis for building any friendship. As defined by Tony Robbins, the well known speaker and lifecoach, rapport is a "total responsiveness between two people." Simply put, it is a connection between two people with something in common. Whether meeting someone new at a social event or entering a patient's room for the first time, building rapport is essential. By attempting to maintain a certain air of professionalism, healthcare providers unknowingly become unrelatable, placing barriers to relationship building and preventing trust. Today's patient assumes that doctors, nurses, and medical staff are qualified. However, to build a relationship, patients must first feel a connection. They cannot build rapport with "the doctor" or "the nurse." They can, however, establish rapport with "Dr. Orsini, who is from New Jersey and hates the cold" or "Nurse Cindy, who has two dogs and a teenager who is sometimes challenging." Therefore, it's absolutely essential to find commonality with patients, and no matter what differences two people may have with regards to ethnicity, socioeconomic status, or religion, I believe there is commonality among everyone. Physicians and nurses should start conversations by asking non-medical questions and share personal information about themselves. Of course, I am not suggesting to give patients your address, or social security number, but information about where your family comes from or how many children or pets you have makes you a genuine person.

One of my partners, Dr. Gregor Alexander, whom I've had the pleasure of working with for many years, is perhaps the best example of how building rapport leads to a genuine connection. Gregor has been a neonatologist for over 40 years. It was his hard work and dedication that led to the building of the first state-of-the-art children's hospital and NICU in Orlando. Today, the Alexander Center for Neonatal Care is one of the largest and most prestigious NICUs in the world. Dr. Alexander's name is displayed largely over the door at the entrance. One would expect all of the reverence paid to him would translate into a certain arrogance and superiority and that the parents of the babies he cares for would feel intimidated by him. This expectation changes just a few minutes after the parents meet him. To their surprise, they find a humble man who is honored to care for their baby. He asks them personal questions with genuine interest and he shares something about himself. The nurses who work with him often joke that if you give Gregor three minutes, he will find a way that he is related to any family. In just a few moments, the man with his name on the entrance of the NICU becomes the friendly doctor from Colombia who has lived in Orlando for more than 40 years and loves to come to work every day.

Once a connection is made and rapport is established, a relationship forms quickly. To the patient, you become a real person who has a life outside the hospital. You are suddenly perceived as a friend. The patient's emotions will be lightened. They will feel less vulnerable. And if something does not go as smoothly as hoped, they will be more understanding. After all, it is hard to be mad at your best friend.

As healthcare workers, we are privileged to information that the general public is not. We know which physicians are clinically sound. Yet, the most talented physicians are not always the ones with the most successful practices, and most of us can name several great clinicians who struggle to attract patients. The difference is that the physicians with thriving practices are better able to build rapport with their patients and create loyalty.

Before she died, my mother-in-law was treated for many years for a leaky heart valve that required at least two major surgeries. Her cardiologist, Dr. Isaac Winthrop, was an old-timer who did not always keep up with the latest medical literature or use the newest medications. Nevertheless, he had a thriving practice for many years. One day, after my mother-in-law was admitted to the hospital for the third time in one year, I suggested that perhaps she should consider going to a larger university hospital and get a second opinion from another cardiologist that I knew had an impeccable reputation for being the best. She immediately dismissed my suggestion with contempt, sharply answering, "I could never change doctors." "Why mom?" I asked. She answered without hesitation, "He is so nice. Whenever I go to his office, he shows me pictures of his grandchildren." To her, it didn't matter whether or not Dr. Winthrop was the best cardiologist or that she may have received better care somewhere else. Dr. Winthrop was her great friend and she would remain loyal.

Here is another example of how being genuine can help build rapport and make patients and family feel valued. It is now well accepted that daily rounds by the nurse managers of the hospital are a real patient satisfier and I highly recommend rounds at least once a shift. However, it's crucial to remember that it's not just about the act of rounding, it's how they are done that's important. In other words, it's all in the delivery. It is how the nurse manager interacts with patients during patient rounds that will determine whether or not a connection is made. For instance, most of the nurse managers whom I observe entering a patient's room will say something like, "Hi, Mrs. Smith, my name is Francine and I'm one of the assistant nurse managers on the floor. I'm doing my daily rounds and I wanted to see if you needed anything." The problem with this approach is that it seems forced and sounds like a script. When patients are asked if "they need anything," it is interpreted as a shallow request hoping that the answer is no. The patient's perspective is that the manager doesn't really care and she is only asking because it's her job. The patient is merely a checkbox on a to-do list.

But manager rounds can be meaningful and serve as a real opportunity to establish rapport. A better approach would be to say, "Hi, Mrs. Smith. My name is Francine and I'm the nurse manager on the floor today. Nurse Lydia tells me that you are doing well, but I like to get to know all of my patients, so if it's okay with you, I'd like to sit and talk for a minute." In this example, the patient believes that the nurse manager genuinely cares. Mrs Smith feels that Francine really wants to get to know her as a person—it is not forced. Since Francine is visiting because she wants to and not because she has to, Mrs. Smith is much more likely to ask questions and tell her what she needs to make her more comfortable. A relationship has been formed almost instantly.

Smile with Your Eyebrows

There is nothing better than a smile to begin a conversation and make someone feel welcome. However, how we deliver a smile can also make a big difference. Smiles come in all shapes and sizes and can be interpreted very differently. For instance, smiling with just your mouth is perceived as shallow and insincere (and maybe a little creepy). Add some facial expressions and it becomes warm and heartfelt. Many have heard the term "smile with your eyes." Using your eyes when smiling elicits a feeling that you are genuinely happy to see the other person. It doesn't appear to be forced. Raising your eyebrows during a smile takes smiling to a whole different level. It states nonverbally that you recognize the person as a welcomed friend.

Here is a fun thing to do the next time you are at work or at a public place such as a supermarket. Find someone that you have never met, smile with your eyebrows raised and say hello. Then watch their response. Almost always, the person will feel as if they know you and respond with a very similar smile.

Why is smiling with your eyebrows such an important skill for clinicians to learn? Typically, a doctor has hundreds of patients in their practice and it would be very difficult to remember each of them with any depth. Greeting your patient while smiling with your eyebrows evokes familiarity and makes the patient feel that you remember exactly who they are and that you are excited to see them. For any healthcare provider, this technique is a great first step towards building rapport.

Principle #3: Thank God I have a friend in the business.

After 17 years as a practicing neonatologist in the Northeast, I finally convinced my wife to move to a warmer climate. By the grace of God, I was offered a job at Winnie Palmer Hospital for Women and Babies in Orlando. The WPH NICU is a state-of-the-art facility designed to allow parents to live in the same room as their premature babies. Shortly after starting my new position, I experienced what the principle of "having a friend in the business" really meant.

I was working on the 11th floor of the NICU. Typically, the more stable babies stay there and are seen toward the end of the day after the critically ill babies on the 3rd floor are examined and treated. My wife had taken my youngest son TJ to the ophthalmologist for a routine exam. TJ was a freshman in high school and was just starting to acclimate to his new environment. I can recall my exact location on the 11th floor when I received a call from my wife

Lauren. She called to tell me that the ophthalmologist was referring TJ to a specialized eye clinic in Miami for further evaluation. The eye doctor saw a spot on my son's retina and recommended that he be seen immediately by a specialist. Because I'm a doctor, it was fairly easy to get the ophthalmologist on the phone. From one physician to another, I asked him frankly what he saw on my son's retina. We had never met, but I knew right away he was avoiding my question. His communication skills were lacking and he fumbled over his words, desperately trying to get me off the phone without telling me what he saw. He finally gave into my persistence only after it was clear that the conversation would not end unless he acquiesced. He blurted out, "I don't think it's a problem with his retina. I think he has a brain tumor pushing on his eye. I think he should have an MRI as soon as possible."

My whole world stopped at that moment. All of the research I had done on Breaking Bad News, all of what I had taught for years, and all of the interviews with patients about how bad news changes your life forever, was happening to me. I still remember the exact spot I was standing near the bench in the hallway. I couldn't move, let alone ask any more questions. All I heard was brain tumor, referral to Miami, and MRI as soon as possible. Clearly not being trained in the art of Breaking Bad News, the doctor quickly, and not very convincingly, asked if I had any questions and hung up the phone.

As I sat down on that bench, everything went silent. The background noise of the world's largest NICU went away. I didn't hear the alarms or the people who later told me they asked me if I was okay. The next thing I remember was one of my partners who noticed me sitting there, pale and paralyzed. He was shaking my shoulder and asking what was wrong. Dr. Michael McMahan was one of my new partners. He had been at WPH for more than 20 years and knew everyone, not only at Winnie Palmer Hospital but at the children's hospital connected by a walkway across the street. Michael and I became immediate friends when I first arrived in Orlando. He and his wife Sally had the same interests and same aged children, and they were the first friends Lauren and I made when we moved to Florida. Michael is an excellent neonatologist with a big heart and is totally dedicated to his patients. It took a few minutes for me to explain to Michael the news I had just received about my son. Without hesitation, Mike took me across the walkway to the radiology department at Arnold Palmer Hospital for Children. He introduced me to the pediatric radiologist on call that day and explained to her that TJ needed an MRI as soon as possible. The radiologist made a few changes in her schedule and was able to get TJ scheduled at 9pm that evening. This made me feel a little less anxious, but it was still only 3pm.

The MRI was difficult. As with many patients, TJ had trouble staying still. Claustrophobia set in, so we requested that the anesthesiologist come to sedate him. Since TJ's MRI was not scheduled in advance, the anesthesiologist was not available, but once again, I was able to convince the anesthesiologist to make an exception and help TJ get through the MRI. I would need another favor and some more juggling of the schedules before the MRI would finally be completed. The radiologist read the MRI immediately and, thankfully, there was no brain tumor. Later, we learned in Miami that the spot on the retina was nothing more than an unusual birthmark.

TJ was fine. There was no tumor or serious eye defect. But the six hours between my wife's phone call and the MRI were, without a doubt, the longest of my life. If it were not for "having a friend in the business," I can't imagine how I could have waited for days or weeks to find out the MRI results.

Even though I had already been teaching the principles of Breaking Bad News and had seen how patients and families reacted, it was not the same as personally experiencing the potentially tragic news about my son. The experience validated what I had been preaching for years. As with anything in life, whether it's your first time falling in love or biting into a jalapeño pepper or going skydiving, there's nothing like the real experience. No matter how much you read about something or have something explained, the actual feeling only becomes completely real when it happens to you. After the incident with TJ, I understood more profoundly how patients and families feel because I had been in their shoes. I became more devoted to learning about compassionate communication and, ultimately, how to teach others its benefits. The whole experience made me more passionate about my overall mission. I fully understood what it must be like being in a vulnerable position and not having a "friend in the business."

If you're a healthcare professional and you have worked in this field for any length of time, I am sure you have received many phone calls from friends or family members asking for medical advice. Requests for recommendations about a doctor, or to help them navigate through a complex medical system, or even to get treated in the emergency room faster are common. In my case, I was fortunate to receive special considerations through my connections. Because of my friends and colleagues, the nightmare only lasted a few hours instead of days. However, most people experiencing a health crisis do not have an inside connection. Their fears, confusion, and anxieties are, nevertheless, just as real. Therefore, it is vital that we become their friends. In order to truly have a good experience, every patient should feel as if they have a friend in the business. My advice is to make them feel special from the very beginning of your encounter and let them know that you are on their side. Extraordinary experiences come from extraordinary efforts. Friends do a little extra for each other.

There are many ways that we can easily make our patients feel as if they are special and have someone looking out for them. For instance, when you meet somebody and you shake their hand and say "it's very nice to meet you," that is essentially a script. You don't really know if it is nice to meet them or not. You have no idea whether they are a good or bad person. It is simply a routine, shallow greeting that we have been trained to say. By contrast, if you say "It's been really nice meeting you" at the end of the conversation, it is not a script. It is genuine. It means, I have had a discussion with you, I have gotten to know you for a few minutes, I have decided that you are a good person and I am genuinely happy to have met you. I find it fascinating that just by saying "It's been nice meeting you" at the end of a conversation, instead of at the beginning, it will elicit a very different response. This slight change in the routine will make patients and families feel as if they have a friend in the business. And it does not require a particularly long interaction.

As stated previously, the patient experience is the sum of all interactions with both medical and non-medical staff. Therefore, it is essential that everyone who encounters a patient be trained in the principles discussed in the chapter. Here is another example of how a non-medical staff member can make a patient feel special. When a patient calls for an appointment, instead of simply stating, "The doctor is booked. We can't fit you in for an appointment until next Tuesday," a better response is, "I'm sorry, Mr. Johnson, the doctor is booked until next Tuesday. If you can hold on for just a minute, I'll see if I can squeeze you in sooner." Even if the receptionist comes back on the phone and says, "I'm sorry Mr. Johnson, I tried, but I just couldn't squeeze you in. If I get a cancellation, I will personally call you," the patient will appreciate that the receptionist at least tried to get him/her in sooner. And by using the word "personally," they formed a bond with the patient on the phone.

The same is true when a hospital patient is anxiously waiting for the doctor to arrive. The patient knows that physicians are busy and that it's possible that they may have been called away for some emergency. One way nurses can relieve the anxiety of patients is by offering to personally call and see when the doctor is planning to arrive. This type of extra effort and service goes a long way to ease a patient's nervousness and build a bond. With one small gesture, the nurse has become the patient's friend in the business.

Principle #4: Feel. Do not just think.

It's been said that even the most horrible experiences can become the norm if they occur frequently enough. The volume of patients physicians encounter every day lends itself to making even the most severe diseases seem routine. It's common for doctors and nurses to refer to patients by their disease instead of their name: the pneumonia in Room 306 or the lung cancer in Room 410. In today's fast-paced, economics-driven medical environment, it's easy for the busy doctor or nurse to become task-oriented instead of patient-oriented. We surrender to the pressure to move faster and see more patients, forgetting the human side of medicine. The only solution to this trap is to use our imagination and place ourselves in the shoes of the patient. Without imagination, true compassion can never be achieved. We must remember that what is routine for us is not routine to the patient. For instance, Ms. Jones may be the fifth person this week admitted for appendicitis, but from her point of view, this situation is unique, inconvenient, and possibly quite terrifying.

For most who of us who have chosen the medical field, compassion comes easy when caring for a dying patient or treating someone for a newly diagnosed cancer. It's the patient with the minor illness, however, that's often ignored and is the first to fall victim to routine care. We need to remind ourselves frequently that patients with even the most minor illnesses need our compassion, too. Taking a moment to imagine what our patients must be feeling will allow our compassion to flow.

For example, in any NICU, there is much sadness and much joy. Emotions are high day and night. Although many patients do not survive, the large majority do very well. In fact, most babies admitted to NICUs have short stays and go home healthy. Sadly, many are not so fortunate. Dispersed among the more healthy babies are the micro-preemies (babies who are born less than 26 weeks old) for whom severe complications and/or death are much more frequent. The parents of these critically ill babies sit vigil by the incubator during the day and go home each night terrified they will receive a phone call with devastating news. To the nurses and doctors in the NICU, the focus tends to go toward the critically ill baby who requires more of their time.

Regardless of whether their baby is critically ill or just requires a few days of observation, each parent feels grief. Their hopes of delivering a healthy baby and going home from the hospital in a few days with their son or daughter in their arms have been shattered. They are emotional and feel a lack of control. Some parents handle the stress better than others and each has different needs. The parent of the critically ill patient who is feeling emotional or is demanding is often comforted by the staff. The demanding or emotional parent of the "routine" baby is labeled high maintenance or difficult. Any NICU nurse or doctor can probably recall the desire to bring the "demanding" mother or father of the more healthy baby into the room of the dying baby and remind them that their situation could be a lot worse so stop complaining. Thankfully, I have never seen this actually happen, but I must admit it has crossed my mind and the minds of most of the doctors and nurses I have worked with. Imagination is the antidote to this desire, which is born out of frustration and is intensified by a pressure to perform better and faster. It's a trap that anyone can fall into. The solution is simple. First, you must be able to recognize when it is happening. Be aware when your focus is becoming more about getting work done and less about forming relationships with your patients and families. Then, stop and imagine what it would be like to be that mother in the NICU or the patient who just had surgery. To them, emotions are not dictated by comparing illnesses. Patients and families don't view being sick as a choice between having cancer or appendicitis. Both are extremely stressful.

Principle #5: It is all about relationships.

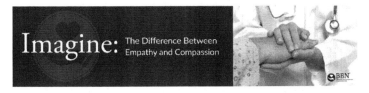

Effective and compassionate communication is the foundation for all medicine. Communication in medicine is not just about accurate information. Too often, the conversation centered around better communication in medicine is pointed toward more accurate records or easier access to laboratory values and consultant notes. Communication in medicine is more than inputting and sharing data. It's more than ensuring that nurses accurately sign out during shift change. Of course, all those things are important, but communication in medicine is most importantly about understanding the needs of the people in our care. It is less about the quantity of information and more about the quality of the communication. The skilled communicator is able to use the principles discussed in this book to form a human to human connection with anyone in a brief period of time. Sharing personal information, being a friend to the patients, and acting in their best interest will give patients a sense that they are cared for and respected. Extraordinary experiences are often the result of the most simple gestures.

Shortly after moving to Orlando, my wife's parents came to visit for an extended stay. They were both in their upper 80s and had their share of medical issues. Within five days of staying with us, both needed to be hospitalized. My mother-in-law was admitted to the telemetry floor on a Monday afternoon, and by Wednesday, a fall required my father-in-law to be admitted to the same hospital just two floors below his wife. On the third day of my father-in-law's hospital stay, the nurse manager came to do her rounds. Practicing good communication skills, she sat with him and asked him a few personal questions. My father-in-law quickly became comfortable enough with her to mention that his wife was in a room just two floors up and that this would likely be the first anniversary that they spent apart in 50 years. Shortly after the nurse manager left, a gentleman entered the room, introduced himself as being part of the transport team, and told my father-in-law that he had been instructed to bring him to the gift shop to buy a rose and then wheel him to see his wife. My in-laws were able to spend a few hours with each other that day and were both released a few days later. For years, neither of them quite remembered why they were in the hospital. They don't remember that there was a two-day delay for the cardiologist to read the echocardiogram. They don't remember if the food was tasty or the hospital was well decorated. What they remembered was that amazing nurse manager who took just a few minutes to find out what my father-in-law truly needed and then did something extraordinary.

As doctors and nurses, we can use our communication skills to not only improve a patient's experience but to ease the pain and suffering as well. Talking to a patient about their interests can take their mind off the pain they are feeling or allow them to forget the anxiety about an approaching procedure. In the book, *First, Break All the Rules*, Gallup reports an interesting study involving exceptionally talented nurses. Working with a large healthcare provider, 100 exceptional nurses were compared to 100 average nurses. Each was asked to give an injection to the same population of patients. Although the injection was given exactly the same, the patients reported feeling less pain from the needles that the exceptional nurses administered compared to the average nurses. How could that be? The technique was the same. The needle was the same size. What researchers found was that it was the manner in which the exceptional nurses spoke with the patients that made the difference. They immediately built rapport. They were able to convey empathy and assure the patients that they would do their best to ease the pain. In a few short sentences, they eased the anxiety of the patient.[38]

Chapter 6
Compassionate Communication and the Well-Being of Healthcare Providers

Anthony Merk, M.D.

Dr. Anthony Merk was my family doctor as well as the doctor for most of the Italian-Americans who lived in the North Ward of Newark in the mid-to-late 1900s. He practiced medicine for over 50 years—so long that he delivered me as a baby and was the first physician I did my clinical rotation with as a third-year medical student. For those who may not be familiar with the schedule of medical school, students traditionally spend the first two years in the classroom. They memorize and recite, attend class for eight hours per day, dissect cadavers, and then go home to study until midnight. The next morning, the routine starts all over again. The students who survive two years of this unforgivable pace are allowed to progress to clinical rotation. Each student spends their third and fourth year completing mandatory and elective rotations in each specialty. This system gives them the opportunity to apply what they have learned in the classroom to real life situations. It also gives the student a very general knowledge of all aspects of medicine and provides them the opportunity to sample each medical specialty before choosing which area to continue their training as a resident.

Dr. Merk also specialized in obstetrics and gynecology. By today's standards, this type of doctor rarely exists. Family medicine physicians now require three years of residency training after graduation and another three years of residency for the additional specialty of obstetrics and gynecology. In 1948, when Dr. Merk graduated from medical school, there was no residency requirement for family medicine allowing a physician who graduated from medical school to immediately apply what he learned to a private practice. However, Dr. Merk decided after graduation to complete a residency training program that would allow him to specialize in women's health, including delivering babies and performing OB/GYN surgeries. It was a good career move considering that in the 1940s the entire OB/GYN training was only one year compared to three years today.

As far back as I can remember, Dr. Merk was old. I guess to a young child, even a 40-year-old seemed like an old man. He dedicated his life to his patients and practiced medicine almost until the day he died in his late 80s. One of the amazing facts about Dr. Merk is that he practiced for over five decades and, to my knowledge, was never sued for malpractice. Many years later, having experienced the litigious nature of medicine, I became increasingly curious how Dr. Merk was able practice for so long and never get sued. Was he a perfect doctor? No one is perfect. Is it possible that he never made a mistake? That is doubtful. He was human. So why, after all those years, didn't any of his patients file a lawsuit against him? As I did more and more research on how doctors communicate, it occurred to me that the key reason was that he had an amazing ability to form friendships instantly with each and every patient even if he was meeting them for the very first time. To those who knew him, no matter how briefly, he was not just "the doctor." He was a genuine person whom they could relate to and trust. He was a person with real life interests, perhaps some flaws, but one who loved what he did.

For me, Dr. Merk was almost part of the family. I suspect all of his patients felt the same way. As such, his patients understood that no matter what the circumstances or outcome might be, Dr. Merk had their best interests in mind. So even if something went wrong, the thought of contacting an attorney or filing a complaint would never be entertained. After all, no one sues a friend.

We looked forward to seeing Dr. Merk at every visit. He always had a smile on his face and asked us about our personal lives. We felt that he was genuinely happy to see us, and looking back, he often smiled with his eyebrows. He had a dry sense of humor and loved to tease and joke with his patients. It put us at ease and we had total trust in his abilities. When we left his office, we felt better even before the prescription was filled. We had total confidence that if anyone could heal us, it was Dr. Merk.

Having looked up to him all my life and thinking of him as an honorary uncle, it was natural for me to choose him as my mentor for my first elective clinical rotation as a fourth-year medical student. Of course, whom else would I choose to spend time with than Dr. Merk? Looking back, I cannot say that I learned a lot of medicine from the old doctor. His medical books were ancient; I used to joke that they were probably original editions. His methods were not always up to date, or even the most evidenced-based. It wasn't until years later that I realized just how much he taught me. By watching him interact daily with his patients, I learned how to greet a patient with a smile, and how to instantly build good rapport and trust. I learned how to make patients feel comfortable even without medicine. I learned that being able to communicate and show genuine compassion toward patients and families is the key to building a successful practice. I also learned the power of humor and how to make patients feel better through laughter when appropriate.

Dr. Merk would smile at his patients when they told him about their symptoms. When he looked at them right in the eyes and nodded, they knew he was listening with real compassion. There was no question in their minds that his attention was on them and only them. It instantly made them relaxed and confident that they were in capable hands. I never saw Dr. Merk multitask. There was no writing in the chart while the patient spoke. In fact, most of his patients' entire charts were kept on a 5x8-inch index card. Dr. Merk's patients were so dedicated to him, that most of the local female patients would always bring him a home cooked meal when they came for their office visit. Homemade spaghetti, eggplant parmigiana, and meatballs filled the refrigerator in his back room. Yes, I must agree that I ate very well during that clinical rotation.

Dr. Merk understood early in his career that when patients and families trust their doctor and believe they have genuine compassion for their situation, they are more likely to follow the prescribed treatment, stay loyal to their doctor, and have better outcomes. This, of course, is now well documented. Dr. Merk seemed to know it naturally. When medical schools were teaching physicians to be scientists and telling them to be distant observers, Dr. Merk taught me how to be a genuine person and build trust. I may have not realized it during my time working with him, but, in retrospect, the lessons he taught me have had a profound effect on my career. He was decades ahead of his time and helped me find extra meaning in my life's journey.

Medical Errors and Malpractice Claims

Despite the best efforts of hospitals to improve the processes in which medical care is provided, medical errors remain one of the leading causes of death in the United States.[39] To address this problem, hospitals have put great efforts to concentrate on standardizing care: using electronic medical records, computerized order sets, and other technologies to reduce human error. These are all important steps toward safety but, unfortunately, have had limited success. Similar to the failed efforts designed to enhance the patient experience, attempts at reducing medical errors have not adequately addressed failures in communication first. According to the Joint Commission on Accreditation of Healthcare Organizations (JCAHO), up to 80% of serious medical errors are attributed to poor communication. This includes communication breakdown between patients and healthcare providers as well as breakdowns between medical staff. To further support the strong relationship between poor communication, medical errors, and malpractice, a 2015 report by CRICO Risk Management Foundation at Harvard University found that 57% of medical error cases reflected miscommunication between two or more healthcare providers, while 55% involved miscommunication between providers and patients. This represents a huge number of cases that could potentially be eliminated if healthcare professionals were trained how to communicate better. If we are to address the crisis of medical errors, we must first provide proper communication training to all healthcare professionals.

It is also important to note that malpractice lawsuits have been directly related to a physician's communication skills. Studies have shown that 71% of malpractice lawsuits are due to communication errors.[40] Learning how to communicate and interact effectively with your patients and families is the best protection against lawsuits. According to the American Bar Association, patients are much less likely to sue their healthcare providers if they have a trusting relationship with their physician, even if they are advised to file a suit by an attorney or friend. Yet, risk management departments and hospital attorneys continue to preach more and more documentation as a method for avoiding lawsuits. The mantra of "If you didn't write it down, you didn't do it" is embedded into every healthcare provider's head from an early stage of training. The demands of more documentation only encourages multitasking. In many cases, physicians and nurses have become so concerned about lawsuits that they forget the patient is a human being and not just a diagnosis. Many have been pushed into treating every patient as a potential lawsuit, resulting in more defensive documentation. "I informed the patient this and told the patient that" or "I checked this and answered all of their questions." Every detail of the visit is documented in the most defensive manner. The words of my medical school professor ring loud in my mind whenever I write a hospital note about a patient. He told us to, "Write the note as if you are speaking to an attorney." Is this what we have become? How could a bond form that starts with the assumption that the patient is the enemy? Without trust, there is no relationship, and the risk of malpractice lawsuits actually increases. It is clear that today's physicians can still learn a lot from Dr. Merk. He needed no more than a 5x8-inch index card for his office notes. It wasn't the documentation that kept him from getting sued. It was the relationships he built. Patients generally understand that doctors and nurses are humans, and by being human, we are imperfect. The truth is, most patients do not sue because of poor outcomes; they generally sue because they have questions that were not answered and don't feel that the care they received was done by someone they trusted.

Communication techniques can be used to predict lawsuits.

Nalina Ambady, a Harvard psychologist published a paper in 2002 examining how the tone of a surgeon's voice can predict malpractice history. In her study, Dr. Ambady recorded audio of surgeons speaking to their patients during routine office visits. At the time of the study, half of the surgeons had previous malpractice claims and the other half had never been sued. Ten-second clips were extracted for each surgeon from the first and last minute of their interactions with two patients. The tone of their conversations was rated by coders blinded to the surgeon's malpractice claim history. The clips were rated and analyzed for several variables including warmth, hostility, dominance, and anxiety. The study found that ratings of surgeon's tone of voice from very brief segments (four, 10-second clips) of audio-taped conversations were significantly associated with the previous malpractice claims toward the surgeons. Even when controlling for content of conversation, the coders could predict the surgeons who had a malpractice history simply by analyzing the tone of the voice. In summary, a simple analysis of a physician's communication techniques can predict malpractice history. It truly is all in the delivery.[41]

Professional Burnout and the Patient Experience

In the healthcare industry, physician burnout has been estimated to be as high as 50%, and recent studies have shown that more than 50% of physicians report at least one symptom of burnout.[42] Worst yet, physicians have the highest rate of suicide among any profession and are twice as likely to commit suicide as the general population. Among nurses, a study by the human resource company KRONOS® HR Solutions reported that more than three out of five nurses (63%) stated that their work has caused job burnout, and two out of five (41%) stated they have considered changing hospitals in the past year because they have felt burned out. Also, 93% said that they felt mentally and physically drained at the end of their shift, and 11% said they frequently left their shift worried that their fatigue led to substandard care. Luckily, hospitals are beginning programs, such as providing access to a psychologist, to help those suffering burnout.

Certainly, there are multiple factors that contribute to this epidemic. Long hours, the threat of malpractice, and the increasing administrative demands are all factors. But we have been sold a bill of goods for more than a century. We have been told by our mentors and medical school professors that in order to protect ourselves from burnout, we must limit our emotions. Medical schools have led students to believe that by practicing "detached empathy," they can avoid burnout. It turns out that, in fact, the opposite is true. Recent studies have shown compassion to be protective against burnout.[24] Why would this be the case? Psychologists have known that when people act in contrary to their core beliefs and values, they feel less fulfilled. Nowhere is this more pertinent than to the medical profession. In 2012, a study of 3,200 Canadian doctors was able to predict who will experience exhaustion and poor work performance by identifying the people whose personal values conflict with the values promoted in the work environment. In other words, when doctors fight their natural tendency to feel compassion by closing off their emotions, burnout is more likely.[43]

I believe that almost all healthcare professionals start out with an altruistic view of medicine, determined to heal the sick and conquer all disease. But the demands on physicians and nurses to document meticulously, and to see a growing number of patients each day coupled with the false narrative that we are better healthcare providers if we stay detached from our emotions, have led us down the path to burnout. Only by recognizing this downward path and learning how to better communicate with compassion can we break this cycle of physician burnout and patient dissatisfaction. It admittedly takes time to master compassionate communication through constant exercise, but in the end, I believe it will reduce burnout and serve our patients better.

Let's look at an example of how burnout develops.

I work at one of the busiest neonatal intensive care nurseries in the country. Systems have been put in place to achieve maximum efficiency while maintaining the highest standard of care. With so many patients to see each day, the computer helps keep track of which babies have been seen by a doctor. The patient's name turns from red to green after the physician or practitioner examines the baby and prints the daily progress note. As is the case in most hospitals or physician offices, the high pace and increased demands of seeing a large number of patients make it very easy for the providers to become task-oriented. In fact, sometimes, if I'm not careful, I can become so task-oriented that I often feel like my job is to turn red to green. This can, and I believe does, happen to almost every healthcare provider at one time or another. What happens next is what eventually leads to burnout. When we become too task-oriented and don't take the time to feel compassion and make that human connection with our patients, we act contrary to our core beliefs and values. This results in decreased job satisfaction, reduced engagement, and even depression. We leave work and feel unfulfilled. Perhaps we are not sure why, but there is a feeling that we did not complete our job, no matter how perfect the clinical medicine might have been. Each day runs into the next and we become more unlike the altruistic idealists that we once were. Over time, this lack of compassion and human connection with our patients causes increasing disenchantment and eventually burnout. I have found that the best way to avoid burnout is to break the cycle. If we can be more aware of when we are becoming task-oriented and spiraling into burnout then we can better protect ourselves and remember the reason we entered healthcare in the first place.

The truth is, the more compassion we allow ourselves, the easier it becomes. There is actually a neuroscientific explanation for this fact. The brain's social communication circuits involve two main structures: the insula and the anterior cingulate. These two structures work together to express compassion and empathy. They are also involved in conflict resolution and the recognition of deception. Studies have shown that the frequent expression of compassionate communication actually increases the size, thickness, and activity of both structures in the brain.[42] Therefore, we should show our compassion frequently through words, deeds, and body language because it is in line with innate human values and enhances our ability to feel compassion, and avoids burnout.

Chapter 7
Conflict Resolution: What to Do When Something Goes Wrong

Even Jesus had enemies. That's what I tell my wife when she gets a less than perfect online review. My wife is a successful realtor and heads a top-notch team in New Jersey that consistently ranks in the top three in sales and ratings every year. Their success is no surprise to me. She has an incredible ability to build rapport with new and old clients, and I have witnessed first-hand the type of service she and her team provide to every client. Answering the phone late at night on a weekend and paying meticulous attention to every detail during each transaction ensures her clients have the best possible experience. She has mastered the five principles of communication discussed in Chapter 5 and her success is proof that they work. She and her team have nearly a 98% rate of positive reviews. Yet, occasionally they receive a less than flattering online comment. This, of course, is unavoidable. No one is perfect. The reality is that, no matter how hard we try to please everyone, there will be an occasional unhappy customer or patient. When that happens, how we handle it makes all the difference.

When it comes to healthcare, the stakes are bigger and emotions run higher. Everything is magnified, making it even harder to reach 100% positive reviews. Patients feel vulnerable and scared and are forced to give up some control of their body to others whom they most likely have never met. No one lies in a hospital bed by choice. They start out unhappy, not with the hospital or doctor, but with their circumstances. When something does not go smoothly in a hospital or at a physician's office, no matter how insignificant, it can result in a high level crisis situation. The reality is that no matter how good our intentions might be or how well we follow the rules of compassionate communication, something will inevitably go wrong. Hospitals are busy places with a myriad of moving parts, personalities, and complex systems. Fortunately, medical errors or substandard treatments are responsible for only a very small percentage of patients who are unhappy or dissatisfied. The overwhelming majority of complaints are due to communication breakdown either between hospital staff or between healthcare providers and patients. Learning the proper communication techniques to form relationships with patients early can bank good will and avoid a bad situation altogether. But when something goes wrong, resulting in an unhappy patient or family member, how the complaint is handled initially will either escalate or defuse the situation.

The Lost Luggage—What Not to Do

Although I grew up in New Jersey and love the people, I always hated the cold weather and dreamed about moving south to a warmer climate. After more than 20 years of hearing me complain about the cold, my wife agreed that if the perfect job opportunity would present itself, she would consider moving to Florida. With a reputation for providing top-notch care for the sickest of newborns, Winnie

Palmer Hospital provided that opportunity. It was a last-minute interview that required squeezing it into my already busy schedule. I was able to find an evening flight with a major airline that I had never used before and will remain unnamed. I arrived at the Orlando airport around 11pm the night before only to find out that my luggage was lost. Panic was my first emotion. I had only nine hours before my interview and all I had to wear were the sweatpants and hoodie sweatshirt that I wore on the flight. I entered the lost baggage claim area to find a very pleasant young lady who greeted me with a big smile. I told her that I had an interview early in the morning and my luggage was nowhere to be found. Her very well meaning response was, "Don't worry, Mr. Orsini, this happens all the time. I will take care of it." Although she meant for her words to be comforting, they had the opposite effect on an emotional, anxiety-ridden, middle-aged physician. My immediate thoughts were, "OMG, this airline loses luggage all the time." Had the young lady understood the concept of "It's All in the Delivery," her statement may have been more encouraging if she told me, "Don't worry Dr. Orsini. This rarely happens, but when it does, I am trained to find it quickly."

I'm not sure if I would have received a job offer if I had shown up for the interview in a sweatsuit, but fortunately, I didn't have to. The airline found the luggage and had it delivered to my hotel before my meeting the next morning. We escaped the cold of New Jersey and have been Floridians ever since. Over the course of my research and experience, I have found that by applying many of the same communication techniques discussed in this book, we can better resolve conflict when approaching an unhappy patient.

The Four Pillars of Conflict Resolution

1.   I have no preconceived notions
        about the situation.

2.   This is very unusual.
        It doesn't happen very often.

3.   I will personally take care of it.

4.   This is your idea, not mine.

Diffusing a bad situation, or as some say, "turning a negative into a positive," can be accomplished if we follow four specific steps. It's what I call the four pillars of conflict resolution as outlined below.

1.   *I have no preconceived notions about the situation.* Very often, when a customer, patient, or employee is unhappy about a situation, the manager is called to help solve the problem. Managers often make the mistake of informing the unhappy person that they have already investigated and have the facts before hearing their side of the story. The intention is meant to tell the them that, as the manager, he/she took the time to prepare and is taking the situation seriously. Unfortunately, this has the opposite effect. Telling an unhappy patient or customer that you already know the facts before allowing them to tell their story suggests to them that you have spoken to your team, have already de-

cided that you know who was right, and are simply there to deliver a message of unity with your team member. In this situation, patients are unlikely to give a thorough explanation of what happened and why they are upset. Feeling that you have already determined that they are wrong only makes them more angry. Alternatively, telling the unhappy patient that you have minimal facts with no predetermined ideas about the problem will help the patient stay calm and encourage them to speak and be heard. I am not suggesting that you don't obtain the facts before entering the conversation with the patient. Just don't let them know. All that is required is that you keep an open mind before speaking with the patient and not give the impression that your decision has already been made.

For example, enter the room and say, *"Hi, my name is Susan, and I am the nurse manager in charge. Jennifer tells me that you wanted to discuss a problem with me. She wasn't specific but I'd like to find out more so I can help."*

This tells the patient that Susan has no preconceived notions about the problem and is ready and willing to hear what the patient has to say. It is also important to remember that an angry patient or family member is most likely, under these circumstances, upset and prepared for an adversarial conversation. Don't immediately address the situation at hand—take a moment after introducing yourself and ask non-medical questions. Don't immediately get to the point. Use the communication techniques covered in the previous chapters to build rapport. This will go a long way to diffuse the situation. Use your body language to de-escalate the situation. This is a great time for sitting down casually with legs crossed and a smile. Share something about yourself and make that genuine connection first. Then, discuss the circumstances behind the complaint. Using this technique, you will likely calm the patient's family down and, by building rapport first, you will better be able to diffuse the situation quickly. Let's improve upon Susan's technique even further.

"Hi, my name is Susan, and I am the nurse manager in charge. I like your New York Yankees hat. Are you from New York originally? I am also a baseball fan, but my team is not doing that great this year. Jennifer tells me that you have a concern about your care. She wasn't specific, but I'd like to find out more so I can help."

In this example, Susan quickly builds rapport first by building a relationship with the patient before addressing the problem. In my experience, this is the most effective strategy for beginning any conflict resolution.

2.   *This is very unusual. It doesn't happen very often.* Despite our best efforts, there are many moving parts in a busy hospital or medical office. It is difficult to predict how long it will take for test results to come back or when a consultant may be able to visit the hospital after long office hours. Delays and minor mishaps happen more than we would like to admit. It's important that no matter how common this occurs, the staff does not make the same

mistake that the young lady in baggage claim made when my luggage went missing. Telling a patient that delays or problems "happen all the time" is not comforting. It further aggravates the situation by adding to the emotional doubt the patient is already feeling. No one wants to place their health and their well-being in a hospital that experiences delays and mishaps all the time.

3.   *I will personally take care of it.* The best relationships are made on a one on one, human to human basis. It is impossible to have a trusting relationship with an inanimate object, such as a hospital, or a vague group of people collectively known as "we." After listening to a patient or family, and describing the uniqueness of the situation, give a guarantee that you will "personally" take care of it. There are, of course, situations that are beyond the control of any one person. For instance, we cannot guarantee that a consultant will be at the bedside by a certain time or that a test result will be back immediately. We can, however, guarantee that we will personally try our best to make it happen. The words bond that patient to the one making the promise. It puts a face to the person responsible for rectifying, or at least attempting to rectify the situation, and instantly creates a relationship. Instead of being assured that someone will call the consultant's office to get a timeline for his visit, use the words, "I will personally call." It will almost always de-escalate the situation and assure the patient they are in good hands.

4.   *This is your idea, not mine.* A comedian once polled

his audience to find the couple who had been married the longest. When he asked who had been married for more than 50 years, one couple raised their hand and was asked to stand up. The comedian asked them to share their secrets of a successful marriage. The gentlemen promptly answered with a loud voice and proud chest, "She makes all of the little decisions and I make all the big ones."

"That's very interesting," the comedian replied. "What would be an example of a big decision?"

The husband quickly answered, "I am not sure, we haven't had one yet."

For 50 years, the wife was making all of the decisions while still allowing her husband to feel pride that he was in control. The point of the story is simple: if you lead a horse to water, he will decide to drink, but if you tell him to drink, he may not choose to. For the most part, disagreements occur when two parties see things from their unique perspective not realizing that there is another way to view the problem. This is the essence of the fourth pillar of conflict resolution and what "It's All in the Delivery" is all about. When a customer or patient is upset about something that did not go smoothly, instead of giving explanations of why it occurred and giving your recommendations on how it should be resolved, bring the unhappy patient along with your thought process as you troubleshoot the problem. If done correctly, more often than not, the patient will come to the same solution or conclusion as you did, giving them a sense of control that they so desperately need.

Chapter 8
Putting It All Together

Andia and Keith Kolakowski were a young couple in love, excited about having a baby and, like most couples, anxiously waiting for the big day their son would arrive. They did everything right, reading books on pregnancy, preparing the baby's room, and eating healthy. By all accounts, the pregnancy was going well and their excitement was growing. Suddenly, at 23 weeks gestation, Andia experienced sudden onset of preterm labor. Despite attempts to stop the labor, Andia delivered her son Isaac 17 weeks early. I met Andia and Keith briefly before their baby was to be delivered and explained the dire situation. Although the chance of survival for their baby was low, they prayed for the best. Isaac Kolakowski was born on May 15, 2017, at 1 lb. 3 oz. Only Andia and Keith could possibly understand their joy muffled by feelings of helplessness and pure fright. Andia and Keith sat vigil next to Isaac's incubator. They watched skilled nurses and staff paying meticulous attention to every detail of Isaac's care and felt the warm support of everyone around. My partners and I monitored Isaac closely and applied every bit of the more than 200 years of accumulated experience to help him survive. Despite all of our efforts, on the 15th day, Isaac suffered a severe intestinal complication commonly experienced by extremely premature babies. Isaac went for emergency surgery to repair his intestine but the next day, he died in his mother's arms. Family members and staff were present as doctors and nurses supported the parents during the worst time of their life—sharing tears with the family.

Miracles happen every day. I know, because I see them all the time. I watch as doctors, nurses, and hospital staff perform life-saving procedures and comfort families and patients in the most compassionate manner. As a neonatologist, I practice medicine on the very fringes of life and sadly, despite all efforts, babies sometimes die. It is during these incredibly difficult moments that I also see the natural compassion of incredible men and women. Deep below the layers of hospital administrators demanding efficiency, attorneys threatening lawsuits, and risk managers asking for more documentation, are medical professionals who have dedicated their lives to comforting the sick and most vulnerable. Rabbi Kushner once defined the distinction between curing and healing: "Curing makes a problem go away. Healing means giving a person the resources to deal with a problem that isn't going away." That day when Isaac passed away, the miracle of healing was everywhere.

One would fully expect Andia and Keith to be angry about the death of their beautiful son Isaac. I would understand any parents who may be bitter at the staff or God for not curing their baby. But I have found that the opposite is often true. Family members appreciate the dedication of the medical staff and their efforts and feel an instant bond with the doctors and nurses who grieve with them.

This is where the real miracle of medicine happens. This

human connection lies within us all and is most exposed during difficult times. At its core, healthcare is about a group of human beings applying their knowledge and compassion to help those who can't help themselves. It is the most personal thing we will ever experience.

I found out later that Andia and Keith were both gifted writers. Andia contacted me several months later and told me how appreciative they were of the brief time they spent with Isaac. They wanted to give back to the hospital that gave them time with Isaac and help others who may find themselves in a similar situation. In their words, Isaac entered and exited this earth like a meteorite, making a huge impact in the brief time he was here. Andia and Keith have produced a photo-journal book to help parents with sick babies document the time they spent at the hospital sitting with their babies. *Catching Meteorites* is now in print. The purpose of *Catching Meteorites* is to tenderly care for the mental and emotional health of parents affected by trauma by inviting them into the healing space of guided visual storytelling. It is funded through charitable donations and is given free to the hospital where Isaac lived and died.

Donations can be made through their website: *www.catchingmeteorites.com*

Throughout this book, we have discussed the deficiencies in healthcare, which have resulted largely from poor communication. Medicine has lost its way. Advances in technology, pressure to be more efficient, and attempts to improve the patient experience by erecting bright, shiny, new buildings have misled us into forgetting what medicine is is truly about—one human being comforting another. It is a relationship.

The resources that the sick and most vulnerable need lie in the special bond between patient, family, and medical personnel. Unknowingly, we have been pushed into a task-oriented model at the expense of compassion. But in Isaac's case and in other similar tragedies, I have learned to step back and observe the natural compassion that flows outward during these horrible moments. Suddenly, other tasks seem less important. Team members help each other, clergy is called to the bedside, and the needs of the parents and family become the only thing that matters.

It is my belief that medicine is broken, not because of the people who dedicate their lives to healing but because of the way the current system has forced providers to lose the essential personal connection with their patients. There is a cure, however, and it starts with relationship building. If you are a medical provider, hopefully, the communication techniques covered throughout this book will give you the tools needed to build instant relationships with patients, remind you of why you entered the healing profession in the first place, and bring out your natural compassion. If you are a patient seeking care, my hope is that this book has empowered you to demand more from your physician or hospital. Communication is the foundation for good medicine and better outcomes.[44] For all of us, learning to communicate in our professional and personal life is a journey that never ends, but it is a journey worth taking.

Chapter 9

Interviews

The following are excerpts from the many interviews performed during the decades of research that it took to develop the concepts discussed in this book. I would like to thank the many patients, family members, and dedicated healthcare providers who freely discussed their experiences.

Lucia—Family Member

"I received a call from the doctor at the hospital. My husband was taken there the night before. I was home with the kids when the phone rang. The doctor just said, 'He has an aneurysm'. I kept thinking, aneurysm in the heart? And then he said, 'No, it's in the brain.' I thought I was going to die. I remember I was standing up against the wall. I still had pajamas on. I felt like I was just going to fall to the floor. It's complete shock. You have no physical control of your entire body. And it's not something that takes seconds to go away and you can say to yourself, 'Okay, this is the news that I was given, now get yourself together.' Because you need to respond. It doesn't happen that way. It's a very long process. I don't think they (physicians) understand the impact they have on how it is said. They really need to realize that the parent is no longer just a parent or a spouse but a patient, too.

"Ten years later, my son was diagnosed with leukemia. This time, I was pleasantly surprised. This doctor was so kind. His

mannerisms, his tone of voice, his compassion was something I will be grateful for forever. Even though I had just met him, I immediately felt like I was with someone that I trusted. I felt like someone really understood how I felt."

Nancy—Registered Nurse

"My mom had been diagnosed with breast cancer. It had metastasized basically throughout her body. The day I heard the news was pretty difficult for me to hear the message being delivered. There was one physician in particular who was extremely blunt. He was very matter of fact about it. He just basically walked in and said to me that 'there is nothing else we can do for her and to put her on dialysis would be a huge waste of time on your part. So that's basically it. That's all we can do for her.' I was so angry and asked him to leave. As a nurse, I knew he was right, but don't deliver the news in a 15-second speech and walk out of the door. That was really rough. The families of these patients will always remember the exact moment they got that news and how it was delivered and how they felt. I believe that they pull that into their grieving process.

"The second doctor who came to my mother's room was very different from the first. He really did take the time. He came to my mother's bedside. He sat down with her and held her hand and said 'If you were my mother, I could never have you continue to do this. I know you are in a lot of pain, and if you want to go, it's okay.' It was so heartfelt and I will forever be grateful to him."

Patricia Eaton, D.O.—Board Certified Pediatric Emergency Medicine Physician

"Participating in Dr. Orsini's Breaking Bad News program sort of brought me back to why I wanted to be a doctor in the first place, which I've always been very aware of. But being an intern, I got really busy and caught up in the crazy schedule. But I love medicine, and I love the children. The truth is, I really did come to medicine to be in a specialty and to be a part of people's lives and really be able to talk to them. And I want to be able to make that bad situation as good as possible for parents. The communication training I received gave me the tools to do that. I am forever grateful, and now I teach the same techniques to my residents."

Amy Matherne, M.D.—Board Certified Pediatrician

"I actually had to break bad news as an intern. It was my second month as an intern; I had to break bad news to a parent and I didn't know what to do with myself. The attending (senior physician) was there and I did the best I could and, thank goodness, she was there to jump in when I needed her. One thing I remember, and I get it now, but I didn't at the time, was that she was quiet and she didn't say anything. And I kept thinking, why isn't she consoling him? Why isn't she doing something like telling him something to make him feel better? I get it now that I've completed the Breaking Bad News training. I understand. The one thing that I definitely took away is that silence is important sometimes, just to let the parents go through the emotions."

Bob—Family Member

"I was 20-something, got in my car, drove to the hospital and I said, 'I'm here to see my mom.' The nurse just looked at me, pointed at the room, and said, 'She's there, she's dead.' It's funny, that was more than 20 years ago and I still remember it as if it was yesterday."

Judith—Patient

"I was arriving there (the hospital) showing pregnancy, wearing maternity clothes, excited about a baby. And within five minutes, my whole world had changed and I was leaving the office, despondent, alone, and unsure of what to do next.

"If the doctor had told me that you should really bring your husband, I think I really would have come into the office holding his hand, you know, really prepared to hear some bad news and I also would have been able to ride in the passenger seat on the way home."

Jose Perez, M.D.— Board Certified Neonatologist and Medical Director

"The training program designed and administered by Dr. Orsini has significantly improved the way our physicians, nurses and team members communicate with our families. The ability to measure this improvement using Press Ganey scores, allows us to link staff improvements to financial performance."

Gaines Mimms, M.D.—Board Certified Neonatologist

*"If the family can go away with that feeling that you did ev-
erything you could possibly do, you reached out in a way that
they could understand it. You don't increase their pain. They'll
always have the sadness over the loss or over a diagnosis, but
if they feel that, in some way, that it was a shared experience
and they knew you connected with them at some level, that will
become a very positive experience."*

References

1) Cuddy, A.J.C. (2015). Presence: *Bringing Your Boldest Self to Your Biggest Challenges. Large print edition.* New York, NY: Little, Brown and Company, Hatchette Book Company.

2) McKinley, T., et al. (September 2017). *Burnout and Interventions in Pediatric Residency: A Literature Review.* Burnout Research, Vol. 6 (pp. 9-17).

3) Campbell, J., Prochazka, A., Yamashita, V., and Gopal, T.R. (2010). Predictors of persistent burnout in internal medicine residents: A prospective cohort study. *Academic Medicine* (pp. 1,630-1634).

4) Pantaleoni, J.L., Augustine, E.M., Sourkes, B.M., and Bachrach, L.K. (2014). Burnout in pediatric residents over a 2-year period: A longitudinal study. *Academic Pediatrics* (pp. 167-172).

5) Osler, W. (May 1889). Valedictory address, University of Pennsylvania. Retrieved from *http://medicalarchives.jhmi.edu:8443/osler/aequessay.htm.*

6) Fox, R., and Lief H. (1963). Training for "detached concern." *The Psychological Basis of Medical Practice.* New York, NY: Harper & Row.

7) Blumgart, H. (1964). Caring for the Patient. *The New England Journal of Medicine* (pp. 449-456).

8) Lee, F. (2004). *If Disney Ran Your Hospital: 9½ Things You Would Do Differently.* Bozeman, MT: Second River Healthcare Press.

9) Naykky, S.O., Phillips, K. A., et al. (2019). *Journal of Internal Medicine* (pp. 34, 36-40).

10) Doyle, C., Lennox, L., and Bell, D. (2013). Systematic review of evidence on the links between patient experience and clinical safety and effectiveness. *British Medical Journal.* Retrieved from https://bmjopen.bmj.com/content/3/1/e001570.

11) Groopman, J.E. (2007). *How Doctors Think.* Boston, MA: Houghton Mifflin.

12) Finlay, I. and Dallimore, D. (June 22, 1991). *Your Child is Dead. British Medical Journal, Vol. E.* Retrieved from https://www.bmj.com/content/302/6791/1524.

13) Baile, W., et al. (August 2000). *The Oncologist.* Retrieved from https://theoncologist.onlinelibrary.wiley.com/doi/full/10.1634/theoncologist.5-4-302.

14) Orsini, A. (2018). Get with the PROGRAM: A Guide to Compassionate Communication. *The Journal of the American Osteopath Association* (118 [10], pp. 679-684).

15) Kushner, H. (1981). *When Bad Things Happen to Good People.* Anchor Books (ISBN: 1-40000-3472-8).

16) Lieberman, J., and Stuart, M. (April 1999). The BATHE Method: Incorporating Counseling and Psychotherapy into the Everyday Management of Patients. *Primary Care Companion, Journal of Clinical Psychiatry* (1[2], pp. 35-38).

17) Wolf, J. (2018). *Consumer Perspectives on Patient Experience.* The Beryl Institute.

18) White Paper Consumerism: The Role of Patient Experience in Brand Management and Patient Acquisition. *Press Ganey* (December 2013).

19) Centers for Medicare and Medical Services. *HAHPS Fact Sheet. CAHPS Hospital Survey* (August 2013; Updated September 2013). Retrieved from https://www.hcahpsonline.org/.

20) Betts, D. (2018). *The value of patient experience. Hospitals with better patient-reported experience perform better financially.* Deloitte Consulting LLP.

21) Jha, A.K., et al (2008). Patient perception of hospital care in the United States. *New England Journal of Medicine* (359: pp. 121-131).

22) Zolnierek, H.K.B., and DiMatteo, M.R. (2009). Physician communication and patient adherence to treatment. A meta-analysis. *Med Care* (47: pp. 826-834).

23) Vincent, C.A., and Coulter, A. (2002). Patient safety: What about the patient? *BMJ; Quality & Safety in Healthcare* (11: pp. 76-80).

24) Thirioux, B. and Birault, F. (2016). Empathy is a protective factor of burnout in physicians. *Frontiers in Psychology* (7: pg. 763).

25) Wolf, J. (2017). *The State of Patient Experience 2017: Return to Purpose.* The Beryl Institute Benchmarking Survey. Retrieved from https://c.ymcdn.com/sites/www.theberylinstitute.org/resource/resmgr/benchmarking_study/2017_Benchmarking_Report.pdf.

26) Ashworth, M. (January 2016). Antibiotic prescribing and patient satisfaction in primary care in England: Cross-sectional analysis of national patient survey data and prescribing data. *British Journal of General Practice* (66 [542]: e40-e46).

27) Perspectives on American Health Care. *Press Ganey 2011 Pulse Report.*

28) Hutchinson, B., et al. (2003). Patient satisfaction and quality of care in walk-in clinic, family practices and emergency departments. The Ontario Walk-In Clinic Study. *Canadian Medical Association Journal* (168: pp. 977-983).

29) Chang, J.T., et al. (2006). Patient global ratings of their health care are not associated with technical quality of their care. *Annals of Internal Medicine* (144: pp. 665-672).

30) Farley, H., et al. (October 2014). Patient Satisfaction Surveys and Quality of Care: An Information Paper. *Annals of Emergency Medicine, Vol. 64, No. 4.*

31) Florida Association of Hospitals. Retrieved from https://www.fah.org/fah-ee2-uploads/website/documents/FAH-white_paper_report_v18_-_final.pdf.

32) https://www.heathgrades.com/content/patient-sentiment-report.

33) Hospital healthcare research (August 2013). Retrieved from http://www.hcahpsonline.org/files/August_2013_HCAHPS_Fact_Sheet3.pdf.

34) Rogers, R., and Monsell, S. (1995). The costs of a predictable switch between simple cognitive tasks. *Journal of Experimental Psychology: General* (pp. 124, 207-231).

35) Rubinstein, J., Evans, J., and Meyer, D.E. (March 1994). Task switching in patients with prefrontal cortex damage. Poster presented at the meeting of the Cognitive Neuroscience Society. San Francisco, CA: Abstract published in *Journal of Cognitive Neuroscience*, 1994, Vol. 6.

36) Crenshaw, D. (2008). *The myth of multitasking: How doing it all gets nothing done.* Wiley Press.

37) Swayden, K.J., et al. (2012). Effect of sitting vs. standing on perception of provider time at bedside: A pilot study. *Patient Education and Counseling 86* (pp 166-171).

38) Buckingham, M., and Coffman, C. (1999). *First, Break All the Rules: What the Worlds Greatest Managers Do Differently.* New York, NY: Simon & Schuster.

39) Makary, M.A. (2016). Medical error: The third leading cause of death in the U.S. *British Medical Journal* (353: i2139).

40) Huntington, B., and Kuhn, N. (April 2003). *Baylor University Medical Center Proceedings* (16[2]:pp. 157-161).

41) Nalini, A., LaPlante, D., Nguyen, T., Rosenthal, R., Chaumenton, N., and Levinson, W. (2002).*Surgery* (132: pp. 5-9).

42) Shanafelt, T.D., Hasan, O., Dyrbye, L.N., Sinsky, C., Satele, D., Sloan, J., and West, C.P. (December 2015). Changes in Burnout and Satisfaction with Work-Life Balance in Physicians and the General U.W. Working Population Between 2011 and 2014. *Mayo Clinic Proceedings* (90[12]: 1600-13.Doi: 10.1016/j.mayocp.015.08.023).

43) Newburg, A., and Waldman, M.R. (2012). *Words Can Change Your Brain.* New York, NY: Penguin Group.

44) Lee, T.H. (June 22, 2017). How U.S. Health Care Got Safer by Focusing on the Patient Experience. *Harvard Business Review: Web.*

One of the greatest and most common criticisms of modern medicine is that physicians and health care providers communicate poorly with their patients. To my mind, no one has ever addressed these medical shortcomings as directly and as clearly as Anthony Orsini, D.O. In both the seminars that he has given across the country and now in his book, "It's All in the Delivery," Dr. Orsini teaches all health care providers how to become increasingly more effective, more efficient, and more thoughtful. I am incredibly impressed with what he has done and feel strongly that his book should be mandatory reading for all medical students, nurses, and other providers during their training. More experienced clinicians will greatly benefit from Dr. Orsini's teaching as well. This book represents ground-breaking work that will serve anyone well throughout a career in medicine.

Alan R. Spitzer, MD

Formerly, Director of
Research, Education, and Quality
MEDNAX, Inc./ Pediatrix Medical Group
Sunrise, Florida

Former Chief of Neonatology and
Chairman Department of Pediatrics
Thomas Jefferson University
Philadelphia, Pennsylvania

As a patient with a chronic illness, navigating through a complex healthcare system can sometimes be frustrating. Dr. Orsini's book has shed new light on how patients and doctors should communicate. His engaging storytelling combined with practical tips on how to communicate with my healthcare providers have given me new insights and empowered me to take more control of my own health. I wish this book was available when I first became sick.

MJ Buckner

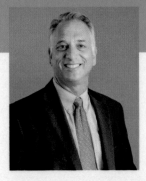

Anthony J. Orsini, D.O.

Dr. Orsini has been a practicing physician for over two decades. He is currently the level II medical director of one of the largest Neonatal Intensive Care Units in the world and serves as chief of patient experience for his neonatal practice. Dr. Orsini has spent the last 25 years developing proven techniques that teach healthcare professionals how to effectively and compassionately communicate with patients. His training programs are used by hospitals and private practices around the country. Dr. Orsini has lectured extensively and has authored several papers on the topics of communication in medicine, enhancing the patient experience and delivering tragic news.

ISBN 978-1-09830-447-8

9 781098 304478